Thai Massage with
Neuromuscular Techniques

of related interest

Tui na
A Manual of Chinese Massage Therapy
Sarah Pritchard
ISBN 978 1 84819 269 0
eISBN 978 0 85701 218 0

Intention and Non-Doing in Therapeutic Bodywork
Andrew James Pike
Foreword by Ged Sumner
ISBN 978 1 78775 898 8
eISBN 978 1 78775 899 5

Cupping Therapy for Bodyworkers
A Practical Manual
Ilkay Zihni Chirali
ISBN 978 1 84819 357 4
eISBN 978 0 85701 316 3

Thai Massage with Neuromuscular Techniques

A PRACTITIONER'S MANUAL

SLAVA KOLPAKOV

Foreword by Dr Richard Gold

SINGING DRAGON
LONDON AND PHILADELPHIA

First published in Great Britain in 2022 by Singing Dragon, an imprint of Jessica Kingsley Publishers
An imprint of Hodder & Stoughton Ltd
An Hachette Company

1

A CIP catalogue record for this title is available from the British Library and the Library of Congress

ISBN 978 1 83997 055 9
eISBN 978 1 83997 056 6

Printed and bound in Great Britain by CPI Group

Jessica Kingsley Publishers' policy is to use papers that are natural, renewable and recyclable products and made from wood grown in sustainable forests. The logging and manufacturing processes are expected to conform to the environmental regulations of the country of origin.

Jessica Kingsley Publishers
Carmelite House
50 Victoria Embankment
London EC4Y 0DZ

www.singingdragon.com

Contents

PART 2: PRACTICE

This book is dedicated to all healers whose aim is to deepen the art of traditional therapies and continue practicing and preserving the healing art of Thai Massage.

Acknowledgements

I owe the making and completion of this book to several individuals who have been instrumental in inspiring me in my healing work and personal life as well as carrying out the nitty-gritty of putting all the pieces of this project together.

To my wife, Theresa, who manages to lend an equal measure of her love, supportive energy, and a critical eye to all my endeavors; and our son Valentin, for his endless joy and brilliance and for making me laugh every day.

To my parents, Nina and Yuri, who have put me on this holistic path early on by teaching and role-modeling the virtues of caring, curiosity, and positivity.

To all my teachers, especially Dr Richard Gold, for his continuous open-hearted support, Jack Baker, for his original teachings of neuromuscular therapy and his editorial help in the neuromuscular portion of this book, Joel Sheposh, for opening the doors to the diversity of techniques of Thai Massage, Koji Hiroshige, for transmitting his passion for the healing arts and the focus of a Samurai warrior, and Masters Pichest Boonthumme and Jack Chaiya, for sharing their wisdom, experience, and being the teachers of teachers.

To Gerhard and Alex Gessner, for letting me use their peaceful yoga sanctuary, the Prana Yoga Center in La Jolla, CA, that is featured in this book in the photos, and for their endless support and friendship.

To all my friends, especially Marie Ahern, for her humor and honesty, and Avery Kretschman, Ann Joseph, and Katrinna Jasso, for their positive energy, willingness to help at short notice, and sharing turmeric lattes.

Foreword

Prior to my first trip to Thailand in 1988, I had never even heard of Thai Massage. At that time, I was the president of a prominent massage school in San Diego (the International Professional School of Bodywork) that offered Chinese Tui Na and Japanese Shiatsu in addition to a full curriculum of Western-style massage and bodywork. I had already been a licensed acupuncturist for 10 years and had done advanced studies in China, Taiwan, and Japan. I mistakenly thought I was fully aware of East Asian styles of bodywork and massage. I went to Thailand primarily to pursue my interests in meditation, yoga, and, of course, Thai food.

Was I in for a pleasant surprise!!

Soon after I arrived in Chiang Mai in the north of the country, I saw a notice for 'Ancient Thai Massage' on the back of the driver's seat of a Tuk Tuk, the wonderful motorcycle taxis that are prevalent in Southeast Asia. On the spot, I changed my plans, I pointed to the sign and asked my driver to take me to receive my first traditional Thai Massage. This literally turned out to be a life-changing decision.

In less than a year, I was back in Chiang Mai to study this traditional style of healing bodywork at the Old Medicine Hospital, at that time, one of only two government-approved schools in the entire country.[1] Combining elements of assisted stretching, yoga, acupressure, and meditative mindfulness, Thai Massage is a unique and effective form of hands-on healing.

As a student, I took copious notes, shot video and still photos, and received numerous sessions of the work at the school and at various massage establishments in the city. At that time, the only teaching materials were simple line drawings. The material was taught in a traditional manner by teacher demonstrations and with no specific references to physical anatomy.

Before returning to San Diego, I arranged for my primary teacher to come to the United States to help establish Thai Massage. Along with others in the West, this turned out to be a stunning success, as evidenced by the remarkable growth and awareness of Thai Massage over the past 30 plus years.

In 2004, Slava Kolpakov enrolled in my Thai Massage program. He clearly stood out as an outstanding student with a keen interest to learn and excel. In addition, Slava also studied neuromuscular and sports bodywork. These

---

1   http://thaimassageschool.ac.th

styles of bodywork emphasize anatomical specificity and provide an excellent therapeutic complement to Thai Massage.

Slava is the perfect person to synthesize and merge two seemingly disparate styles of bodywork that have very different cultural and historical origins. Slava himself is a fascinating combination of origin and influences. He was born and raised in Siberia. He was taught yoga and meditation at a young age. He was a member of the Russian national gymnastics team from ages 9 to 15. In his early 20s he met an American woman in Australia during an ecological study program. He came to America to attend college. Ultimately, this woman he had first met in Australia became his wife. He came to California to study massage and bodywork. He moved to Boston to build a career. Through practice, study, and teaching, he successfully created a synthesis of neuromuscular bodywork and Thai Massage. With this synthesis, he created a new, effective, and profound form of healing.

Now, with the publication of this book, he makes available a systematic, step-by-step teaching manual that is an excellent addition to the growing literature of natural hands-on healing.

Critical concepts are explained that are comprehensive, detailed, and easily understood. Precautions for safe practice are emphasized. This includes tips that help ensure the health and wellbeing of the recipient as well as the practitioner.

This book includes specific Neuromuscular Therapy applications for different muscles and common myofascial conditions and sports injuries. These modules are interspersed within the Thai protocol at appropriate places that are very helpful clinically when treating specific injuries.

One of the great and lasting joys of being a teacher is to witness the growth, evolution, success, and contributions to society of our former students. I am thankful to Slava for providing me with this fulfilling experience.

Dr Richard Gold[2]

---

2 Author of *Thai Massage: A Traditional Medical Technique*, San Diego, CA.

Introduction

During my years as the founder and director of the East West Massage Center, a massage clinic in Boston in the United States, I had the privilege of working every day with a variety of clients of all ages and abilities. Our focus at the Center was always on therapeutic massage applications in sports and injury treatment. We worked with professional athletes around New England, athletics teams at Harvard, Yale, and Columbia Universities, and Boston College, and people with all types of injuries. Because of the breadth of that experience I have been able to apply Thai Massage techniques in those settings and have become adept at identifying and treating injury patterns, whether athletic or otherwise.

This style of therapeutic Thai Massage has evolved over several years of my practice and teaching Thai Massage courses in San Diego and Boston, beginning in 2006, after my return from Thailand.

In Chiang Mai, I attended a number of Thai Massage schools and studied privately with several renowned teachers. Additionally, I received daily bodywork and took notes after those sessions. Toward the end of my studies, I had five notebooks full of stick-figure drawings of techniques: what to do, how to do it, for what condition, as well as what not to do.

Once back in the United States, I had put to the test all the methods and techniques that I had learned. Some of the techniques proved ineffective, repetitive, and even physically uncomfortable. I had to modify and experiment, combining styles and incorporating my knowledge of anatomy, yoga therapy, Neuromuscular Therapy (NMT), and Russian Manual Therapy, which is a type of musculoskeletal therapy. By 2010, I had developed a unique style of my own, which included at least six different schools of Thai Massage and other manual therapy methods.

In addition to the therapeutic focus of this book, I have also chosen to include transitions. By themselves, techniques are like notes without a song, or pearls without a necklace. Fluid logical transitions string these techniques together into a true healing art. When techniques flow from one to the next, Thai Massage is beautiful to watch, just like a dance routine or a Tai Chi form. It takes great practice to acquire the confidence and eventual mastery to blend these techniques into your own sequences that not only feel natural to perform but also, more importantly, serve to benefit the receiver.

Layers

There are multiple layers of learning and performing Thai Massage.

First comes the form. Practitioners must learn how to move their own bodies safely and efficiently through common techniques and transitions. Learning the basic flow is vital in the beginning. This is why most Thai Massage schools teach a specific protocol. Practitioners must get comfortable in their own body and apply good biomechanics in all positions.

Concurrent with the form, it is equally important to know basic musculoskeletal anatomy. As the ancient adage goes, "Above all do no harm." Practitioners must know where to place hands, elbows, feet, and other tools to perform Thai Massage safely and effectively.

Finally come multiple layers of therapy. Depending on their training, practitioners may use various techniques to treat specific conditions. I have chosen to use neuromuscular techniques in my work. However, you may choose other styles and incorporate them into the framework of Thai Massage. Many practitioners combine Chinese acupressure points and meridian stretches with Thai Massage.

Additionally, it is essential to understand different health conditions (for example, sciatica, rotator cuff injuries, lower back pain, etc.) in order to treat them. I will make the assumption in this book that readers will do their own research to be familiar with different conditions when I address them in my treatment protocols.

Patterns

In any art form, there are basic foundational steps, or truths, that stand unchanged. It is what makes an art an art form. The form, or a template, is used to teach beginners. Layers of depth and complexity are added over time, as students assimilate the basics and progress to more advanced stages.

When learning a style of dance or a musical instrument, the student first learns the basic steps, or notes. They learn to see the basic patterns of the art. Step by step. Note by note. Over time, the patterns become more complex, and the student learns to distinguish an increasingly more and more intricate set of patterns within the basic patterns. Patterns within patterns.

Similarly, in massage and bodywork, the body and its movements can be seen as basic steps or patterns. After some hands-on experience, the practitioner will begin to perceive deeper and more subtle degrees of mobility in their clients' joints, pick apart individual muscle fibers and tissues, and sense the flow of energy, whether it is free-flowing or blocked. Therapists must keep in mind these concepts of **layers** and **patterns**, and not rush their natural process of learning. An art is mastered over thousands of hours of practice.

The Origins of Thai Massage

The origins of Thai Massage are hidden in the distant past. Any definitive source on the origins, if even one existed, was destroyed during the many wars between Thailand (then Siam, or the Ayutthaya Kingdom) and its neighboring Burma between the 15th and 19th centuries. The Burmese had sacked, burned, and pillaged the main cities and villages of Siam at least a dozen times, destroying most of the traditional Thai artifacts, records, and writings, which were usually stored in temples.

Nevertheless, the practice of Thai Medicine and Thai Massage persevered in the hearts and hands of the people, as it was passed down from teacher to student for hundreds of years.

The most common historical theory claims that the origins of Thai Massage can be found in northern India at the time of the Buddha around 500 BCE. Massage and manual therapy were indeed practiced by local folk healers in conjunction with herbs, orthopedic medicine (bone setting), breathing exercises, intestinal cleansing, and meditation instruction. However, these healing practices are indeed as ancient as the human race, and clearly predate the Buddha and his contemporaries. Hands-on healing has been practiced since the beginning of humankind.

Thousands of years ago, in every village, in every tribe, there was a place where warriors would go to nurse their wounds, where field workers soothed their aching muscles, and where women gave birth. A medicine woman, or a shaman, provided the healing. In every ancient culture, on every continent, we find evidence of these healing practices.

At the time of the Buddha, hands-on healing was a well-respected trade. It was deemed sacred and kept secret except for the initiated few. The teachers passed their knowledge only to those students who had been vetted as they had shown a certain predisposition, a familial bond, or a natural gift for the healing work.

No doubt that the Thai Massage tradition derived from these ancient roots. As a student of this art, you have the privilege of carrying the torch and paying homage to the tradition and its founders, wherever they may have lived and practiced. It may be in your ancestral heritage, in your DNA, or in your karmic bonds, whether you come from Asia, Europe, Russia, Africa, or the Americas, to become the next lineage holder of this ancient tradition.

The Father Doctor

In Thailand, it is believed that a certain man by the name of Dr Jivaka Kumar-baccha was the founder of Traditional Thai Medicine. He is revered as a saint, an awakened soul, on par with the Buddha, and affectionately referred to as the "Father Doctor." You can see his statuettes on the altars in many people's homes in Thailand.

According to legend, Dr Jivaka was a renowned healer and a personal physician to the Buddha and the Buddhist community in northern India. It seems that he never actually left India and had no direct connection to Thailand.

As an infant, he was left in a basket near a palace, found by the village folk, and brought to King Bimbisara. The king adopted the baby as his own and named the baby Jivaka, from the Sanskrit word *Jiva* (a living being), because the child lived despite having been abandoned.

Jivaka grew up in the palace with other royal children and chose to become a physician from an early age. He studied under a renowned teacher. After seven years, the teacher gave him a test: "Go out into the country and bring back any object that cannot be used for healing." Jivaka traversed the land through and through, healing folks as he passed their villages, and eventually returned, empty-handed. He hung his head as he told his teacher that he could find nothing—everything had some healing quality. He passed the test!

On his way home, he provided healing to people and his fame spread. When the king fell ill, Dr Jivaka treated him successfully and was granted the title of the Royal Physician.

When the Buddha became recognized as a spiritual leader, Dr Jivaka was called to treat the Sangha, the spiritual community. He performed surgeries, mended bones, and administered cleanses, including several cleanses for the Buddha himself.

The story of Dr Jivaka comes to us from *Tripitaka*, an early Buddhist text. There is no mention of massage being used in any of Dr Jivaka's treatments. How his healing work jumped borders and was adopted as Thai Medicine centuries later is unclear. We can only speculate that Buddhism and traditional medicine were brought to Thailand by wandering monks.

Centuries Later in Siam

Buddhism was brought to China around 150 CE, Japan in the 5th century, and to Siam and Laos in the 12th century. As the Buddhist teachings spread across Asia, traveling monks and missionaries brought other practices with them: cultural customs, spiritual philosophy, yoga, new foods, herbal knowledge, and possibly the hands-on healing techniques.

At the time of the Buddha and Dr Jivaka, Thailand as a country did not exist and the ethnic Thai people did not live in that area. Instead, these lands were inhabited by early Khmer kingdoms and other native tribes. It was these early people who were influenced by the Buddhist monks and their practices, combining their native traditional medicine with the arriving knowledge.

Centuries later, around 1000 CE, Thai people migrated from the Guangxi area of southern China. They brought with them the knowledge of Traditional Chinese Medicine. Most likely, this is when the merging of these multiple medicinal practices took place (**Diagram 1**).

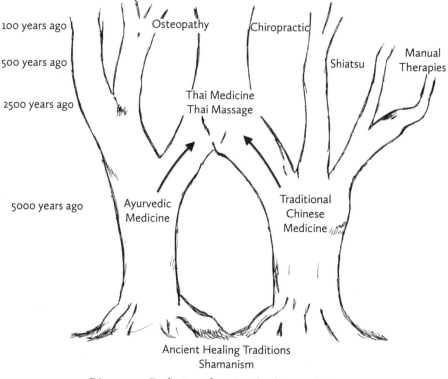

Diagram 1. Evolution of ancient healing traditions

The earliest documented evidence of Thai Massage is from the Ayutthaya period (1350–1767 CE). Remaining Royal Court archives document the existence of a department of Thai Massage (Nuad Boran) organized to serve the Royal family. A French ambassador to Siam wrote in his memoirs in 1687: "In Siam, when someone fell ill, the person with massage experience would start to stretch the body and step on the receiver..."

After the fall of the Ayutthaya Kingdom in 1781, King Rama I implemented measures to improve the overall health of Thai citizens and preserve traditional Thai medical practices. He ordered an old temple in Bangkok (Wat Photaram), that had been salvaged from the destruction of Ayutthaya, to be renovated and to serve as a repository of medical knowledge. In 1832, King Rama II ordered Wat Photaram Temple to act as a university for medicinal arts. Traditional Thai Medicine flourished in the following decades.

This temple is known today as the Wat Pho Temple, where people come from all over the world to learn Traditional Thai Massage.

Branches of Traditional Thai Medicine

- Herbal medicine (including diet and herbal steam baths).

- Orthopedic medicine (bone healing and bone setting).

- Midwifery.

- Thai Massage (including herbal poultice application).

PART 1

THEORY

Being a Healer

I will not rescue you. For you are not powerless.
I will not fix you. For you are not broken.
I will not heal you. For I see you, in your wholeness.
I will walk with you through the darkness as you remember your light.

Sheree Bliss Tilsley, Medicine Woman's Prayer

Thai Massage is part of the energetic paradigm common to all Eastern methods of medicine. It is believed that healing happens when a practitioner becomes an open channel for the Universal Energy, Qi, Chi, or Prana, to flow through them.

The approach varies on the culture it comes from, but generally, the practitioner prepares their energy in the following way:

- Setting the intention of healing before each session.

- A calm and selfless attitude during the session.

- Cultivating an overall body–mind state of wellness ("walk the talk" and "practice what you preach").

It is believed that healing may occur "by osmosis," where the healer's own energetic vibration is so strong and harmonious that it is contagious to their clients.

It is also believed that Universal Consciousness is infinite and omnipotent. Hence, healing may occur at any time, even before the session, especially when both the practitioner and the client set the right intention. It is not uncommon for a client's condition to improve or resolve entirely when they show up at the healer's door. As vessels of this Consciousness, we cannot pretend to know it or understand it. We may only bear witness to the miracles of healing, and life itself.

Thai Medicine Prayer

The Thai Medicine Prayer is chanted individually or in a group in the beginning of each day to invite healing energy into the treatment space. Led by the head teacher or therapist, practitioners bow at the end of each refrain. Additional Buddhist prayers are often included.

(Leader) Handa-Mayan Buddhasa Bhagavato
    Pubbabha Ganamakaram Garoma-Se

(All) Namo Tassa Bhagavato Arahato Samma Sambuddhassa [3 times]

Om Namo Jivako Silasa A-Hang Karuniko
    Sapasatanang Osatha Tipa-Mantang Paphaso Suriya-Jantang Komarapato Paka-Sesi Wantami
    Bantito Sume-Taso Arokha Sumana Homi [3 times]

Piyo-Tewa Manussanang Piyo-Proma Namutamo
    Piyo-Naga Supannanang Pinisiyang Nama-Mihang Namo-Puttaya Nav-on-Navien Nasati-Nasatien
    Ehi-Mama Navien-Nawe Napai-Tang-Vien
    Navien-Mahaku Ehi-Mama Piyong-Mama Namo-Puttaya [1 time]

Na-A Na-Wa Rokha Payati Vina-Santi [3 times]

English translation:

Bowing deeply to the Blessed One, the Worthy One, the Awakened One.

We invite the spirit of our founder Doctor Jivaka.
    May you bring to us the knowledge of nature and healing.
    May this prayer invoke the true medicine of the Universe.
    We honor your guidance and pray that through our bodies you may bring wellness and healing to the body of our client.

The Goddess of healing dwells in the heavens high while mankind stays in the world below.
    In the name of the founder, may the heavens be reflected in the earth below so this healing medicine may encircle the world.

We pray for the one we touch. May they find happiness and illness be released from them.

What You Need to Practice

- A Thai Massage mat, ideally 80 inches long by 60 inches wide by 2 inches thick. Thai Massage mats are usually wider than Shiatsu mats. It is possible to get by with other types of mats such as exercise mats or mattress covers, but these are only temporary replacements and may not be comfortable for your knees and people's backs and hips.

- A Thai Massage mat cover—it is easier to wash a cover than a mat.

- Two long pillows (rectangular), one for the head, and the other for the knees in side-lying position.

- A stack of sheets.

- A stack of hand towels.

- A bolster (optional), for ankles in prone position.

- A heating pad (optional). This is a nice touch in colder months or climates. I prefer to use a Far Infrared (FIR) amethyst-crystal mat.

Before and During Treatment

- Show respect with a bow—Wai Kru (see below). Give thanks to all your teachers, your lineage, before each session. Bow deeply within your heart.

- Let go of selfish thoughts and invite the Universal Energy to work through you. Let yourself relax and trust that what happens is exactly what is needed.

- Listen to the recipient's body. Stay connected to them. Notice where you are guided.

- Maintain a positive mental attitude. Avoid anything that may disturb your mind and clear thinking on the day of your healing work.

- To relax, concentrate on relaxing your abdomen, hands, and jaw. Prior to each session, quiet your mind and breathe slowly into your abdomen and the heart center for several minutes.

- Stay hydrated.

- Learn to breathe evenly and soundlessly during bodywork.

General Body Mechanics Principles

- Whenever you can, position yourself behind your work. Push forward and pull back from your center. Do not twist your spine.

- Whenever you can, lean, melt, and pour. Do not muscle your techniques.

- Work smarter, not harder, by keeping your body as relaxed as possible. If you feel that you are straining and working too hard, you are probably doing it wrong. Reposition, or change your technique.

- Keep your spine as upright as possible. Practice Lazy-Cat Back (see **Body Positions for Practitioners**).

- Keep straight lines in your knees and elbows when performing compressions: 90-degree angles in your arms and legs when palm pressing, kneeling, and foot walking.

- Keep your shoulders loose. Allow your shoulders to "collapse" when palm pressing.

- Thai Massage is like dance. It is not static, but rhythmic, even if the rhythm may slow to the rhythm of the breath. Maintain consistent rhythm by rocking back and forth and side to side. Pour your body weight in and out: emptiness to fullness to emptiness.

- As in yoga practice, do only what is comfortable for your body. If it is not comfortable, skip it. Never perform a technique (no matter how cool you think it is) if it causes pain to you or your client. If you don't know for sure, do not do it.

- Don't know what to do—pray (Thai joke). But seriously, it is okay to ask for guidance from the Greater Power, the Universal Energy, and remain open to it.

- *"Get set, then go."* Do not perform a technique *until* you are physically comfortable. Steady posture is essential. Position yourself first—get set, then GO!!!

- Visualize what you are going to do before doing it.

Body Positions for Practitioners

The following are the most common positions. Although these are the classical positions, there are many variations on the theme. Your body type, joint mobility, and prior injuries will determine your comfort. Some of these positions may not be comfortable at first and may require some practice.

Hero Pose

Vajrasana, or Seiza position, is one of the most common ways to sit in many Asian cultures. I call it Hero Pose for simplicity. It requires good flexibility in the ankle and knee joints. Practitioners sit back on their heels.

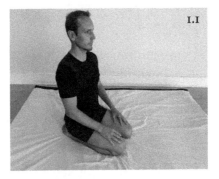

Hero Pose with toes under

People pray in this position in Buddhist temples. However, for many Westerners, this position is torturous for extended periods of time. Ease your way into it, increasing your comfort gradually. This position may help prevent plantar fasciitis.

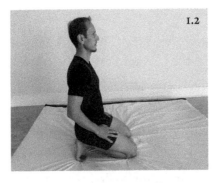

Low Tripod

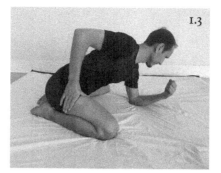

This open-hip position is generally safer for those who have knee discomfort. It minimizes tension in the back muscles as the center of gravity is lower, which makes it easier to flatten, or sag, the back—a position I call "Lazy-Cat Back."

High Tripod

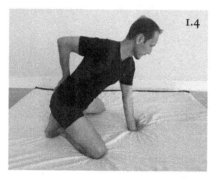

High Tripod provides more leverage/height. It is important to keep the back straight and avoid rounding the back, as in Low Tripod above and Tabletop below. Maintain Lazy-Cat Back.

Tabletop

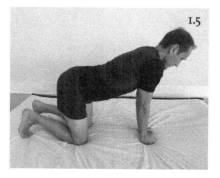

Wide Angle

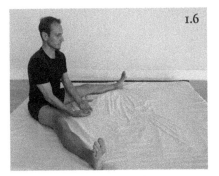

One-Leg-Out

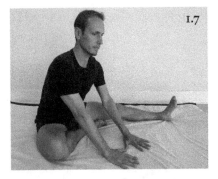

Spiral/90-90 and Sit-and-Lean

The Spiral/90-90 position creates a natural body lean and may be used to perform elbow or forearm compressions. A Sit-and-Lean position leverages the knee to add more weight to the elbow.

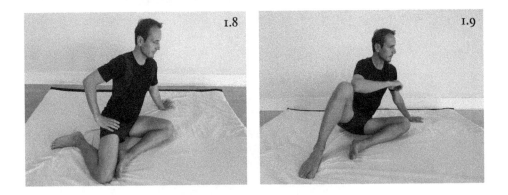

Lunge variations

There are many variations of the Lunge position—wide, narrow, and everything in between.

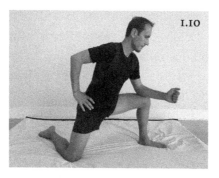

Archer

The Archer is basically a very narrow Lunge. It requires good flexibility in the ankles as the toes are curled under. The upraised knee is used as the tool for compressions and for support.

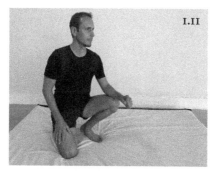

Squat

The Squat is used to leverage one's weight by rocking back and forth in pushing and pulling techniques.

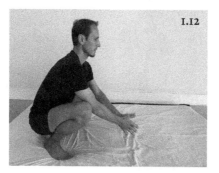

Common Transitions

Performing transitions fluidly ensures a seamless continuity of treatment sessions. Practitioners should aim to keep a fluid rhythm and constant hand contact without breaking their rhythm. There are many transitions that connect techniques together into fluid sequences.

Most transitions are natural and require no explanation as it will be clear from each set of techniques which transition to perform. For example, moving from Hero to High Hero, or Tripod to Low Tripod, or Single-Leg-Out to Spiral, are all one-step transitions and are natural ways to change your body mechanics.

Some transitions may require more than one step. Below are two such common transitions.

Tripod to Archer to Lunge (and back).

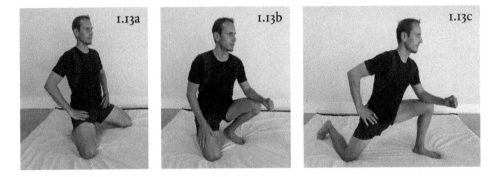

Lunge to One-Leg-Out (and back up the same way). This is easier than it looks. Lean on the arm and fold the bottom leg under.

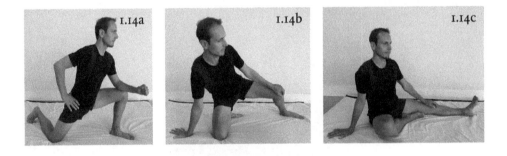

Additional Concepts and Guidelines for Practice

What you imagine is what you touch

If you know anatomy, you can touch specific muscles. If you sense energy, you can address energetic imbalances. Visualization is an essential part of healing work.

Pressure relieves tension

This is a key principle behind all massage and bodywork. We naturally massage or rub an area of pain and tension. This is because pressure provides relief. Gentle pressure is soothing to nerve tissues. Rhythmic pressure flushes out tissues—bringing blood in and toxins out.

Work at the edge

When stretching your client, or performing compressions, take them to "the edge" of comfort—not too little, not too much. Stretching should never be to the maximum tolerable level, and neither should it be too mild. Stretching in Thai Massage is all about lengthening muscles and fascia, and does not need to reach the end of range of motion to be effective.

When shortened, muscles are released more easily

This idea is also behind the practice of Positional Release Therapy and Restorative Yoga. When placed in a supported and slacked position, muscles stop resisting and are able to relax more quickly. During bodywork, bring specific muscle groups into a position of support, and your work will be more effective. This practice does not hold true to fascia, or the connective tissue that surrounds the muscles. Fascia is released better when stretched. Therefore, both shortening and lengthening techniques are needed to be most effective in your treatment.

Use double-point connection

Use two hands, a knee and a hand, or a foot and a hand. Using two points of contact gives the recipient a greater feeling of balance. One hand may feel intrusive. Try to keep several points of connection at all times, so the whole body is involved in treatment. For example, if kneeling, let your knee rest against your client, so long as you are not compromising your own comfort.

Practice precise hand placement

Where do the hands (and the rest of the body) need to be to move from this technique to the next? Paying attention to your own body is essential in discovering your own most comfortable way to move.

Do not overwork the same area

If a client asks for bodywork on a specific area, focus on it for 10–15 minutes, then move away, and come back to it a second time from a different angle or position. Overworking the same spot may cause the tissues to bruise, become inflamed, and go into a spasm.

Clear the Wind Gate points

The Wind Gate points are gates of entry and exit of life force, Prana. When blocked or tender, they signal an imbalance. Clearing these points improves the Prana flow. It is important to clear the Wind Gate points before working on an area, so that energy can move and blockages may be released. Otherwise, stagnant energy may be released from a problem area, but may be unable to exit the body due to blocked Wind Gates. These points will be discussed during the sequence: ankle points, wrist points, points Lu1 and Lu2 under the coracoid process, and point GB20 under the occipital ridge.

Hold deep compressions

Do not move too quickly, and do not pulse or jitter compressions. It is usually more grounding and healing to slow down your rhythm. It is better to sink and hold for 3–4 seconds or even 8–10 seconds on each compression. Otherwise, your session may feel too stimulating and frenetic.

Press, pull, and rock slowly and deeply to the bones and to elicit "joint play"

Press to the bones. Visualize the entire skeletal structure as you work. Notice how each movement (especially pulling, pushing, and rocking) affects the entire structure. Even small movements such as toe pulling should elicit a response in the rest of the body. Let the joints articulate within their range of motion.

Vary your tools

Do not overwork your thumbs or palms. These are common tools where practitioners may experience tension and strain from working too much, too soon. Support your thumb with the forefinger. Include knuckle compressions, elbows, forearms, knees, and feet.

Four Steps in a Session

1. Sensing
Sensing begins with the first meeting with the client, looking over the Intake Form, observing, and listening to their complaints and body language. Let your hands develop the sensitivity of touch—feel the tone, density, and temperature of tissues. Perform a gentle range of motion stretches, palm presses, thumb circles, and thumb-chasing-thumb line work.

2. Warming
Once you know what tissues need to be addressed, warm the area by using deeper compressions and circles: palm presses and palm circles. Explore greater and deeper range of motion (ROM) and passive joint movements.

3. Treating
Apply tissue-specific, muscle-specific treatment—focused pressure using thumbs/fingers/forearms/elbows/knees/feet, as well as trigger point therapy, cross-fiber friction, and deep slow stretching of the muscles and fascia.

4. Reintegrating, or "making nice"
Balance the deep treatment techniques with soothing, feel-good compressions and stretches, brush-outs and jostles, or light chop-chop percussion.

Working with Sen Sib (the Ten Channels)

There are ten primary channels out of 72,000 in Thai Massage. These are "sensed" by sensitive and educated touch and are allowed to "shift" depending on the individual pattern of tension. This is why there are differences in the location of the Sen Sib depending on whom you ask—different sources, or schools, of Thai Massage have different interpretations.

This may seem confusing to new practitioners, especially when the Chinese meridians and points are so clearly and unequivocally delineated (see **common acupressure points** in **Diagram 3**). However, personally, after some practice, it had made a lot of sense to me. For example, if I worked on a client's calf muscles and found a line of tension that is not on a Sen line, I would not ignore that tension just because it is technically off the main channel. I would thumb press through the Sen line and then move on to the actual line of tension and treat it as needed. It is important not to be "stuck" in a pattern.

It helps to know that the Sen lines usually run along common muscle groups and fascial paths and correlate to other meridian systems—Chinese Meridians and Ayurvedic Nadis. Their origin is attributed to Dr Jivaka who based this energetic anatomy on the yogic system of Prana energy flowing through the Nadis (energy channels).

In this book, I have chosen not to focus on Sen Sib as the basis of treatment. There are, indeed, other fine books that do that. I would recommend other sources for those who wish to explore the Sen Sib in depth.

Instead, we will use musculoskeletal and neuromuscular anatomy. We shall refer to Sen Sib as a diagnostic tool, that is, working the lines in the "sensing" stage of treatment. For this purpose, we will not concern ourselves with memorizing the specific names, locations, and effects of Sen Sib. Instead, we will refer to the lines as "inside" and "outside" lines, as in **Diagram 2**.

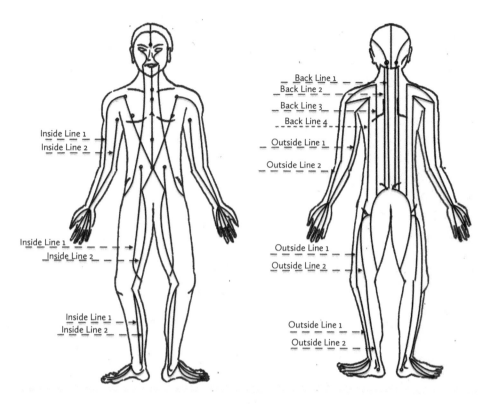

Inside Line 1
Inside Line 2

Inside Line 1
Inside Line 2

Inside Line 1
Inside Line 2

Back Line 1
Back Line 2
Back Line 3
Back Line 4
Outside Line 1
Outside Line 2

Outside Line 1
Outside Line 2

Outside Line 1
Outside Line 2

Diagram 2. The ten Sen lines

Acupressure's Main Points

The following 30 acupressure points (acupoints) are used for treating the most common imbalances (**Diagram 3** and **Table 1**). All these points contain multiple therapeutic benefits. I often use these points to describe a specific location on the body and to correlate with Neuromuscular Therapy's (NMT) trigger points (TPs).

It is important to note that most points are bilateral, unless belonging to one of the two central meridians—CV (Conception Vessel) and GV (Governing Vessel).

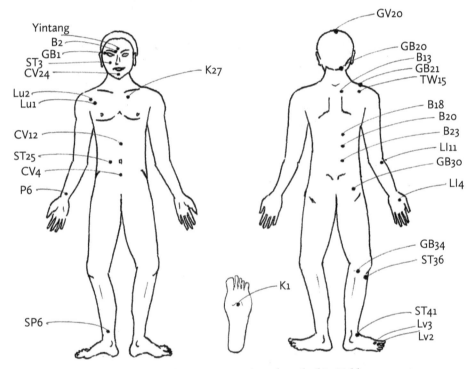

Diagram 3. Common acupoints described in Table 1

Table 1. Common acupoints found in Diagram 3

Yintang (GV24.5)	Third Eye balancing	P6	Relieves anxiety, nausea	Ll11	Relieves arthritis, strengthens immune system
B2	Lowers sinus headaches	SP6	**Super point**, overall regulating, balancing	GB30	Relieves tension in the pelvis
GB1	Stimulating	GV20	Calming, relieves headaches	Ll4	**Super point**, lowers pain overall
ST3	Clears the sinuses	GB20	Treats headaches, tension	GB34	Relieves muscle tension
CV24	Calming	GB21	Relieves fatigue, tension	ST36	**Super point**, lowers fatigue and tension
Lu1	Strengthening for the lungs	B13	Helps asthma, strengthens the lungs	ST41	Opens energy channels
Lu2	Strengthening for the lungs	TW15	Relieves pain, tension in the shoulders	Lv2	Energy reset point, clears blockages
CV12	Aids digestion	B18	Regulates the Liver	Lv3	Treats irritability, low energy, helps digestion
ST25	Aids digestion	B20	Strengthens the Spleen	K1	Revival point, stimulates Chi
CV4	Strengthening, balancing	B23	Strengthens the Kidneys	K27	Wake-up point, relieves anxiety

Thai Massage and Neuromuscular Therapy

This is the crux of the matter, the bee's knees—this combination is the focus of this book and my work in general.

Thai Massage offers a wide range of musculoskeletal techniques to address muscle tightness and joint mobilization issues. Neuromuscular Therapy (NMT) targets the pain and dysfunction in the myofascial system—chronically contracted muscles and fascia entrapping nerve tissues—and the whole neuro-myofascial system gets caught in the infamous Pain–Spasm Cycle.

In the following pages, I will dive into a detailed examination of the principles of NMT and explain how to perform neuromuscular techniques.

Breaking the Pain–Spasm Cycle with neuromuscular techniques

When muscles get shortened and tight, the resulting effects are restricted blood circulation in the area, accumulation of metabolic wastes, and nerve tissue entrapment, all of which cause pain. This muscle tissue pain causes further muscle tension and contraction. In NMT, this cycle is referred to as the Pain–Spasm Cycle (**Diagram 4**).

Nerve entrapment, whether directly by contracted muscles or indirectly by contracted muscles, causing bones to compress the nerve tissue, is a second contributing source of painful input leading to the downward spiral of pain–spasm–pain. NMT interrupts the Pain–Spasm Cycle, improves circulation, and restores normal function in the affected tissues.

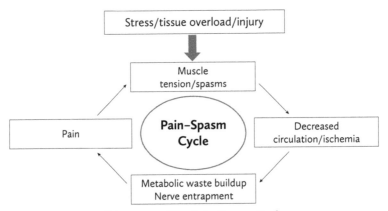

Diagram 4. The Pain–Spasm Cycle

Symptoms of neuromuscular dysfunction or entrapment

- Pain (in muscles, connective tissue, or organs, including headaches and abdominal pain).

- Limited range of motion and stiffness.

- Restricted blood flow (ischemia).

- Poor posture.

- Weakness or loss of strength and function.

- Numbness and tingling sensations (possibly due to pinched nerves).

Causes and sources of pain treated by NMT

There are six causes and sources of pain, as defined by the work of Paul St John,[1] Dr James Cyriax (1982, 1984), and Janet Travell and David Simons (1998).

1. **Postural distortion**

2. **Biomechanical dysfunction**

   These two principles are considered to be the root causes of discomfort, pain, and susceptibility to injury. Examples include rounded shoulders due to shortened pectoralis muscles, or short and tight psoas, causing back pain.

3. **Ischemia** (no or low blood supply to tissues)

4. **Trigger points:** A trigger point (TP) is a point of hyper-irritability that gives rise to pain. TPs develop in areas of ischemic tissue. TPs are both physical (cause changes in the tissue) and neurological (develop a pathological reflex feedback loop, aka the Pain–Spasm Cycle).

5. **Scar tissue or micro-tears:** Scarring in muscles and connective tissues due to visible and microscopic tears is likely to cause pain and impaired function. The scar tissue that forms to heal the tears may cause impairment.

6. **Nerve compression and entrapment:** Chronically contracted muscles may impinge or entrap the nerves that pass around or through the muscle tissue. Osseous structures can also compress nerves. In either case, the result is a painful sensation, loss of strength, and loss of motor control. Release of contracted tissues may relieve the impingement.

---

1   Founder of the Paul St John Method of Neuromuscular Therapy. See www.stjohn-clarkptc.com/paul-st-john-1

Cross Syndromes as Causes

There are two main cross syndromes, described by Vladimir Janda, PT, that indicate muscle imbalances and lead to **postural distortions** and **biomechanical dysfunctions**.

Lower Girdle and Upper Girdle **cross syndromes** describe common patterns of muscle imbalances that stem from poor habits of our modern culture, such as slouching, sitting for long periods of time, staring at closely held devices, lack of walking, and lack of exercise in general.

Practitioners should watch out for these patterns and try to detect these imbalances in clients. Here are some helpful questions to consider when working:

- Which muscles are taut, tight, or short? Which structures may be pulled out of balance by these tight muscles?

- Which muscles are weak? Which structures are not properly stabilized because of the weakness in these muscles?

It is also important to remember that muscles can be weak and tight at the same time. Often, weak muscles become tight in self-protection. When a weak muscle is overloaded, it will contract and possibly stay chronically contracted if not released and strengthened.

The Upper Cross refers to the habitual slouching posture where the pectoralis muscles are too short and tight and overpower the weaker mid-back muscles, while the anterior neck muscles become too weak to resist the jammed-up posterior neck muscles, leading to the forward head posture, as in **Diagram 5**.

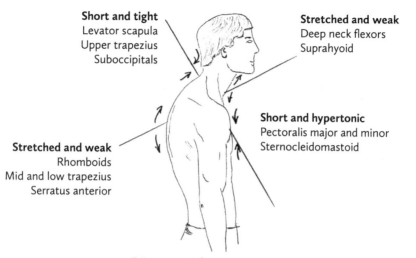

Short and tight
Levator scapula
Upper trapezius
Suboccipitals

Stretched and weak
Deep neck flexors
Suprahyoid

Short and hypertonic
Pectoralis major and minor
Sternocleidomastoid

Stretched and weak
Rhomboids
Mid and low trapezius
Serratus anterior

Diagram 5. The Upper Cross

The Lower Cross shows that our weak abdominals and gluteals lead to the anterior pelvic tilt, pulled forward by the short and tight hip flexor group, thereby jamming the lower back muscles, as in the image on the left of **Diagram 6**. However, lately, with the advent of "chronic over-sitting," I have observed that this Lower Cross has shifted from the tight-weak-tight-weak situation to an all-weak one. The hip flexors are undoubtedly short, but they are also weak from under-use. The back muscles may be short, but they are also incredibly weak and overstretched from sitting too much. This new condition is shown in the image on the right of **Diagram 6**.

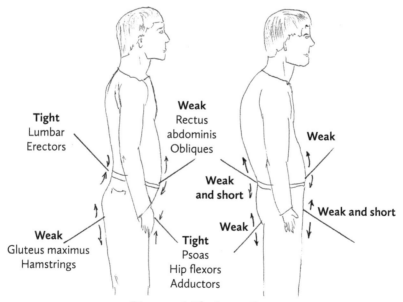

Tight
Lumbar
Erectors

Weak
Rectus
abdominis
Obliques

Weak

Weak
and short

Weak
Gluteus maximus
Hamstrings

Weak and short

Weak

Tight
Psoas
Hip flexors
Adductors

Diagram 6. The Lower Cross

Trigger Points

A myofascial trigger point is a hyperirritable locus within a taut band of skeletal muscle, located in the muscular tissue and/or its associated fascia. The spot is painful on compression and can evoke characteristic referred pain and autonomic phenomena.

Travell and Simons (1998)

Trigger points (TPs) can be found in probably every soft tissue pain syndrome. Referred pain is the distinguishing characteristic of a TP, although the TP itself is not usually painful until you press right on it. The pain referral either spreads out around the TP, or, and this is more common, the referral pattern radiates elsewhere in the body.

The tissues in the area of referred pain may also become ischemic and generate new TPs. Thus, there can be satellite TPs. The pain pattern will continue until the TP is found and treated.

Origins and development of TPs

Travell and Simons present the following theory of TP development (1998). The problem seems to arise with acute muscle strain. The strain overloads the contractile elements in muscle cells, tearing the sarcoplasmic reticulum. The release of calcium ions causes sustained contraction, which requires a constant supply of energy. The area becomes metabolically hyperactive. Nerve-sensitizing substances are also released at the injury site, which causes local vasoconstriction and ischemia. Thus, the pattern is established.

This is a latent TP pattern and causes no pain and draws no attention to itself. It does, however, restrict movement and weakens the affected muscle. Latent TPs can be activated by a variety of acute incidents or chronic stresses at which time they do refer pain and cause irritation. When working on a client, practitioners can find and deactivate both latent and active TPs.

Other factors may predispose tissues to TP development: nutritional deficiencies (B vitamins, vitamin C, calcium, iron, potassium, magnesium), fatigue, anxiety, tension, infection, repetitive motions, and chronic muscle overload.

What to look for

A client can say where the pain is, but not where the source of that pain is. Usually, but not always, a muscle harboring TPs feels tense and the related joint's range of motion is limited.

TPs change the quality of the muscle fibers. Without the muscle actually contracting, palpable bands of fibers around a TP become taut. They feel like *thin needles* lying within the grain of the muscle tissue. If we explore the tissue with a cross-fiber movement (see below), we will be able to distinguish these "taut bands."

Tension builds up around these bands. Often, what we find is more like twine or rope in which the "needles" are embedded. Once such a rope or needle has your attention, explore along its length for the point that triggers the referred pain.

The TP will be an "exquisitely tender" (Travell's phrase) point within the taut band. Clients will let you know, if not verbally, then certainly through their body's reaction. Very often, when you are on a trigger point, the muscle fibers will twitch. The **local twitch response** is a sure confirmation that you are on the right spot.

Another positive indicator of being on a TP is if the client's whole body suddenly "jumps." The so-called **jump response** is completely involuntary and indicative of a TP's location.

Techniques: flat and pincer palpation

There are two ways to locate TPs:

- Use the thumb and fingers like pincers where the muscle allows us to grasp it all the way around—for example, the upper edge of the trapezius on top of the shoulder.

- Where the muscle lies flat on the body and we can only compress into the muscle belly against the firm support of the underlying bones—for example, the infraspinatus.

Client feedback

When you begin to work with TPs, you want to be sure that you find the points and use the right amount of pressure. In the beginning, it is quite difficult to tell where exactly a TP is, and how much pressure is too much. Client feedback can be very useful.

Do not hesitate to ask your client the following guiding questions:

1. Is this point tender or sensitive?

2. Does it refer? Do you feel a painful sensation elsewhere? Or is it in the same spot?

3. Is the referral sensation changing? (Or staying the same?)

When you find what feels like a taut band and perhaps a tiny nodule in the muscle tissue, you want to know if there is any pain associated with this point. Ask if the point is tender, and also determine if the amount of pressure is "okay"—within comfortable limits.

Then, you want to know if the point refers pain when you compress it. In other words, is this point simply ischemic or is it a TP? If there is no referral, you can look elsewhere.

If the point refers pain, and your pressure is within the "good pain" limits, then hold and wait and ask the client to tell you when the sensation changes. You want to know what effect your pressure is having on this TP. If it changes by shifting or diminishing or dissipating—great! If it changes by increasing or getting worse, release your pressure!

The rebound effect

When you are new to TP work, you want to avoid using too much pressure and/or working too long on the same point. This can irritate the point, so the client ends up feeling worse. The best way to work with a TP is with the client's help. Stay within the client's level of comfort, close to the pain threshold.

The tissues may also indicate where that level is because any more pressure elicits the guarding reflex. You can feel the muscle contract to protect itself. That's too much pressure. Some clients will let you go that far, or farther, thinking it is "good for them." It is not!

Hold the pressure constant as you ask the client to tell you when the referred sensation changes. Hold for 10–15 seconds. If the referral doesn't change within that length of time, your pressure is too strong! It is too much input to allow the neural pattern to change. Try again with less pressure; even the tiniest bit less may make the difference.

If the referral diminishes within the given amount of time, there are two ways to pursue to point. Repeat the 10–15-second method a second and a third time. You will find that slightly more pressure is required each successful time to elicit the referred sensation. Always get your client's feedback. The other possibility is to stay with the point and (just as in Deep Tissue work) follow the point as it diminishes or dissolves into the tissues. This usually takes 60–90 seconds and requires much practice and a great deal of sensitivity to subtle changes in the tissue. This technique is called **ischemic compression** because it has the effect of creating a local ischemia in the tissues. When you release, reactive hyperemia sets in—a fresh influx of blood.

This work can be very intense for clients. Intersperse your TP work with some light soothing and rhythmic palm presses and palm circles that disperse the tensions and "make nice."

Cross-Fiber Friction Techniques

Cross-fiber friction techniques are performed at right angles to the direction of soft tissue fibers. Cross-fiber friction addresses the connective tissue, whether that is the fascial wrappings around muscles, muscle tendons, or ligaments.

Normally, healthy connective tissue fibers follow the alignment of the vectors of force, which helped form them. However, due to overuse, injury, or other stressors, some fibers may branch out in other directions and cause problems with surrounding tissues. Such irregular tissues may restrict the movement of adjacent structures. Scar tissue, while it does patch an injured area, also glues together unrelated tissues, shortens muscles and tendons, reduces mobility, and leads to further injury.

By using cross-fiber friction techniques, we can correct these problems to maintain healthy tissue and freedom of movement.

Imagine if every major structure and organ could be dissolved away, leaving only the connective tissue. What would be left of the body?

In fact, there would be a complete body shape composed of a microscopically intricate lattice work revealing the lines of force that course through this physical form due to gravity and the vectors of muscular effort. The shape of each organ and structure would still be recognizable because it is its connective tissue that frames its form.

Technique 1: Broad and soft cross-fiber friction

Broad and soft compressions across muscles are usually performed with palms, thumbs, or fingers. However, knees and feet may also be used once you develop control and sensitivity in those tools.

As you stroke across the grain of a muscle belly, the fascial sheath is stretched and expanded, fibrous accumulations are broken down, and the muscle relaxes and becomes more pliable.

Scar tissue

In times of injury, connective tissue is central to the body's healing response. Fibroblasts flood the traumatized area with collagen fibers in order to "knit" the lesion (wound) back together. The result is a scar.

Connective tissue is not just a collection of fibers. The form these fibers take is dictated by the forces that pass through them—in other words, by movement.

When we are injured, however, the tendency is to immobilize the structure to reduce the pain. Since there is no movement, the collagen fibers are laid down in a random pattern—patching up the hole as best as they can. Some fibers may even adhere to other nearby structures.

As scar tissue matures, it contracts and pulls on the surrounding tissues, causing local ischemia, reduced mobility, and limited function.

The wound—the torn muscle, tendon, or ligament—has been healed, but other problems will follow because of the scar. Local ischemia can continue to cause pain or even foster the development of TPs. The scar itself causes irritation and friction during movement. The scarred muscle is typically weaker than it was before the injury and has a limited range of motion. Therefore, such compromised muscles are more prone to re-injury at the area around the scar.

Technique 2: Transverse friction

Transverse friction is a very effective way to treat scar tissue, both in its formative phase and/or after it has become established. It is a **cross-fiber technique** that focuses expressly on the lesion, the spot where healing is taking or has taken place.

The practitioner anchors into the overlying soft tissue with a finger or thumb and moves that tissue back and forth across the "grain" on the lesion. The purpose is to break down the collagen fiber bonds that are not aligned with those of the healing tissue.

My NMT teacher, Jack Baker, used to say: "If you can twang it, you can 'tweat' it," as a play-on-words indicative of "treatable" grainy and stringy tissues.

The collagen fibers that are aligned form stronger bonds than those that branch out crosswise. The friction breaks down the weaker fiber bonds. We are, in effect, eliminating those fiber bonds that we don't want (across-the-grain bonds and adhesions).

Technique 3: Light transverse friction

Light transverse friction can be applied to a fresh injury after 48 hours, if the swelling and inflammation have gone down. This type of friction should cause no pain. Light transverse friction is done for only 2–3 minutes at a time, followed by an ice pack, up to six times a day.

As a gentle stimulation, friction helps flush the area and keeps fresh nutrients coming in. Cross-fiber bonds are broken down before they become deeply rooted. Light palming, thumbing, and stretching techniques can be applied.

Technique 4: Deep transverse friction

When the injury is old and the scar tissue is well established, we reach for stronger methods and tools. Deep transverse friction gradually wears away cross-fiber bonds. It frees the tissues for independent movement.

Deep transverse friction can be uncomfortable. Inform your clients of the potential discomfort. A few minutes of light transverse friction (palm circles) should precede the deep transverse friction to habituate the local nerves; 8–10 minutes of deep transverse friction on any one location is enough for a session. The area can be iced again afterward to avoid inflammation and pain. Depending on the injury it may require three to five treatments to resolve the problem.

Contraindications and Areas of Caution

- Acute injury or acute inflammation.

- Bone fractures and joint dislocations.

- Fever from any cause.

- Varicose veins (avoid the area locally).

- Contagious skin conditions (check with the client).

- Drug or alcohol intoxication.

- Cancer (allowed if approved by the physician first; avoid the site of the tumor).

- Ill health (acute heart conditions, stroke, high blood pressure, diabetes).

- Pregnancy (Thai Massage specific for pregnancy is okay).

Table 2 and **Diagram 7** show specific areas of caution or endangerment sites. Note that it is not prohibited and it is, in fact, often advisable to work in these areas (for example, sciatic notch to release the piriformis). However, therapists must be well versed in the detailed anatomy of each area and understand the dangers of compressing the wrong thing.

Table 2. Areas of caution found in Diagram 7

1. Inferior to the ear Styloid process of temporal bone, carotid artery, facial nerve	2. Anterior triangle of the neck Carotid artery, jugular vein, vagus nerve, thyroid gland, lymph nodes	3. Posterior triangle of the neck Brachial plexus nerve roots, subclavian and brachiocephalic arteries, jugular vein, lymph nodes	4. Sternal notch Vagus nerve, trachea
5. Axilla Axillary arteries and veins, brachial plexus nerves, lymph nodes	6. Inferior tip of the sternum Xiphoid process	7. Medial humerus Median and ulnar nerves	8. Central abdomen Aorta—main artery, vagus nerve

9. Floating ribs	10. Cubital fossa Arteries, veins, and nerves—radial, median, and ulnar	11. Femoral triangle Femoral artery, nerve, vein; great saphenous vein, lymph nodes	12. Top of the foot Dorsalis pedis artery
13. Twelfth rib, kidneys	14. Sciatic nerve	15. Popliteal fossa Popliteal artery and vein, tibial nerve	16. Head of the fibula Common peroneal nerve

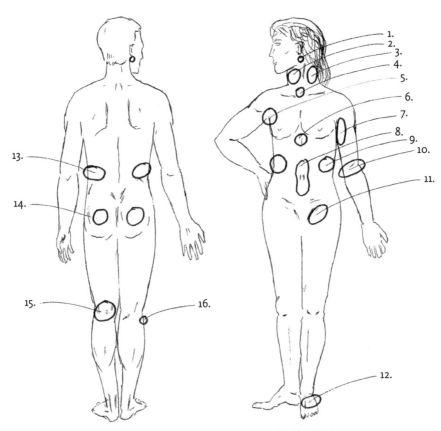

Diagram 7. Areas of caution described in Table 2

Wai Kru: The Bow of Respect

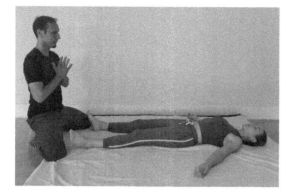

The meaning

With deep respect and love, I bow and ask for guidance from the Buddha.
I bow and ask for guidance from the Father Doctor.
I bow and ask for guidance from all teachers and healers of this tradition.
I bow and ask for guidance from Mother Nature who sustains us.
Let me be a pure and clear channel for the healing energy.
Let me continue to preserve this tradition within my work.
Let me effect a positive change in my client's wellbeing.

PART 2

PRACTICE

Learning the Flow

It is essential to learn the flow of a foundational protocol of Thai Massage. Like learning a new sequence of moves in a Tai Chi form or memorizing the notes of a song, we must first learn the basic flow.

The flow is not the same as the techniques. The flow is everything: the techniques, the positions, the intention behind each move, transitions, rhythm, as well as breathing and mental focus.

The protocol presented here is comprised of traditional musculoskeletal sequences common to all schools of Thai Massage. However, it includes only those techniques that have been found therapeutically viable, or effective, for various myofascial conditions. You will not find potentially compromising techniques as in too-close-for-comfort positions or acro-yoga moves.

The protocol is sequenced in a logical way that eliminates or minimizes complex transitions. Its steps are numbered as part of the flow. When practicing, it is helpful but not necessary to follow the protocol. Practitioners may choose to add other sequences, or skip steps, as they wish.

There are 20 **clinical focus modules** that feature specific Neuromuscular Therapy (NMT) applications for different muscles and common conditions. These are interspersed within the protocol at appropriate places, although they lie outside the basic "flow" protocol. Beginners and less experienced practitioners are encouraged to skip these clinical features for now, while learning the flow, and to come back to them after gaining a working proficiency of the basic protocol.

We pay special attention to body mechanics by including positions and transitions from one technique to the next.

Finally, before we dive into the sequence, it is important to note that this book is only a guide. It is not a substitute for learning Thai Massage or NMT without an experienced and qualified instructor.

Supine—Lower Body

After Wai Kru, we start with the assessment of the body. Our intention is to create balance in the body, improve energy flow, and release myofascial and energetic blockages. Therefore, we check for imbalances, stiffness, soreness, and any other irregularity in the tissues.

Step 1. Sensing

A. Notice the client's passive hip rotation by looking at their foot turnout. Which foot is rotated out more? A greater external hip turnout indicates looser hip flexors on that side, and possibly shorter, and/or tighter, external hip rotators.

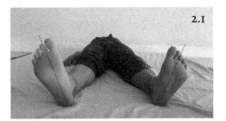

2.1

Position: Hero or Tripod.

B. Take a slow breath in. Place your hands on the client's feet. Exhale, letting your energy connect with their energy field. Take this moment to sense what this individual needs the most: areas of focus, depth of pressure, specific techniques.

Step 2. Palm press the feet

Palm press into the medial arches.

This introductory palm press is like "saying hello" to the body.

Caution: Do not press down; instead, press up toward the head.

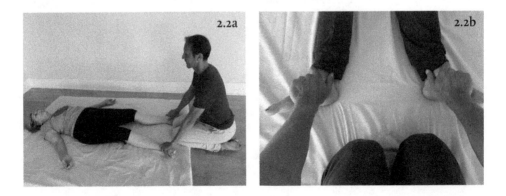

2.2a 2.2b

Step 3. Windshield-wiper ankles

Press at the ankle joint, not on the toes.

Make sure to switch your hands from medial to lateral malleoli.

Compare tension or resistance side to side, checking hip rotation and ankle flexibility.

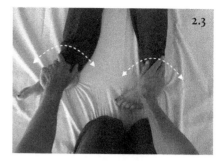

Step 4. Toes-over-toes press

Cross toes over toes.

Press down 3 times—mild–medium–deep, and hold for 3 seconds. Re-cross and repeat.

Transition: Tripod into **Squat** (optional). Curl toes under and roll back.

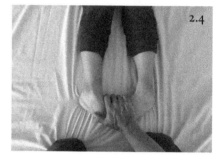

Step 5. Leg traction

Rock back and forth, using your body weight, 4–5 times.

Check leg length by bringing the medial malleoli together.

Place the feet down, shoulder-width apart.

Transition (optional): Squat to **Tripod.**

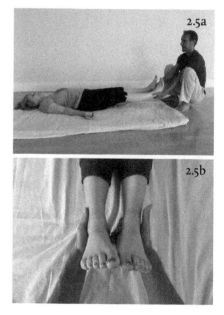

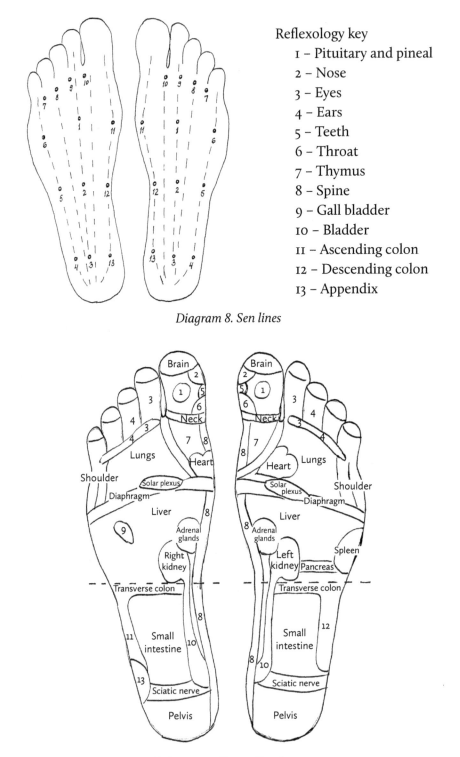

Reflexology key

1 – Pituitary and pineal
2 – Nose
3 – Eyes
4 – Ears
5 – Teeth
6 – Throat
7 – Thymus
8 – Spine
9 – Gall bladder
10 – Bladder
11 – Ascending colon
12 – Descending colon
13 – Appendix

Diagram 8. Sen lines

Diagram 9. Foot reflexology

Step 6. Sen lines press

Thumb press upward to the client's head. Follow points 1–13 on **Diagram 8**.

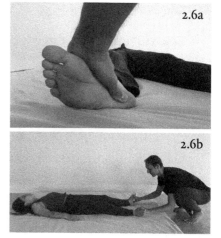

Refer to the **Foot reflexology chart (Diagram 9)** to tone specific organs (press and circle).

Deeper option: If you are still in the squat position, drop your elbows low and brace them against your knees. Press up with your thumbs, rocking your body weight forward.

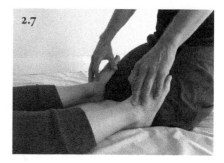

Transition: Squat to **Tripod**.

Step 7. Top of feet finger circles

This technique opens Sen lines on top of the foot.

Walk your knees into the client's feet, to lock them in.

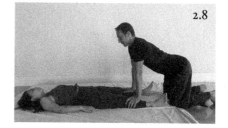

Use all five fingers—press and circle up from the ankle crease to the toe mounts, rubbing over the flexor tendons. Repeat 3–4 times.

Step 8. Lower leg palm press

Palm press or palm walk.

Press directly onto the tibia—keep your palm pressure broad and soft.

Go up and down 2–3 times from the medial malleolus up to the knee and back.

Do not press directly on the knee.

Step 9. Lower leg inside lines

Refer to **Diagram 10**.

Line 1: Thumb walk directly off the tibia, up and down.

Muscles: Posterior tibialis.

Line 2: Thumb walk—up and down—from the posterior medial malleolus along the medial half of the **gastrocnemius** to the knee crease.

Transition: Scoot up closer in **Hero**, or step up to **Lunge.**

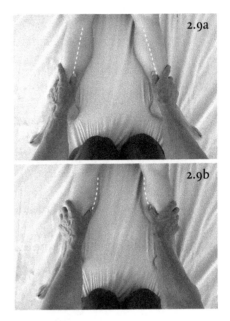

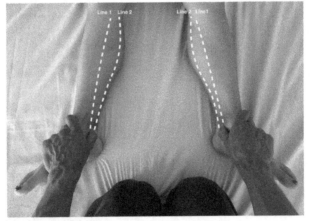

Diagram 10. Lower leg inside lines

Step 10. Kneecap circles

Cup the client's knees with your palms and circle gently to move the kneecaps.

Do not press down hard.

Circle 5–6 times each way.

Transition: Step up to **Lunge** (either side).

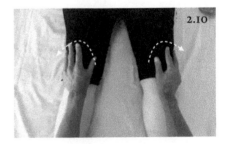

Step 11. Quads and hips palm press

A. Palm walk or palm press, up or down, 2–3 times. Keep your arms straight and use your body weight.

Compress hip flexors and hold for 8–10 seconds.

Muscles: Tensor fascia latae, rectus femoris, sartorius.

B. Quad scoop. Scoop the quads lateral to medial with fingers on the iliotibial band (ITB) area and roll through "the ropes" of the muscles with palm press.

C. Pelvic bowl rock. Keep the center of the palms on the iliac crests/anterior superior iliac spine.

Make sure not to glide or slide on the bones to avoid "skin burn."

Transition (optional): Hero. Bring your knees together and sit back between the client's knees.

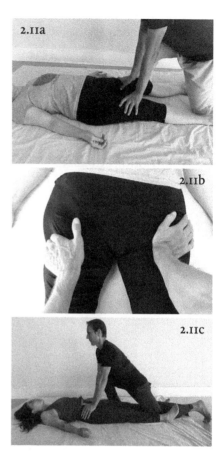

2.11a

2.11b

2.11c

Step 12. Upper legs inside lines

Line 1 (continuous with lower leg line 1): Alternating thumb press—press to the bone (medial-anterior aspect of the femur).

Start above the knee joint and move upward, then downward.

Location: Medial anterior femur, approximately between the vastus medialis and adductor muscles.

Line 2 (continuous with lower leg line 2): Alternating thumb walk—press in toward the bone (medial femur), up and down.

Location: Middle of the adductors.

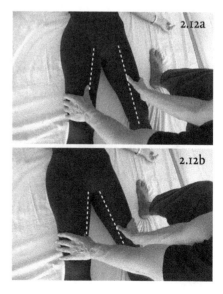

2.12a

2.12b

Transition (optional): High Lunge (back leg straight) or **Down Dog.**

Step 13. Blood stop

Now that the leg energy lines are open, "blood stop" may be performed.

Blood stop is an ancient technique used to improve blood flow in the lower body and to flush out old "sticky, stagnant" blood by first blocking and then releasing the femoral artery (**Diagram 11**).

Contraindications: Pregnancy, high blood pressure, varicose veins, advanced osteoporosis, diabetes. Check with the client before performing!

Good for: Circulation problems, edema in the legs, numbness and neuralgia in the legs, low back pain.

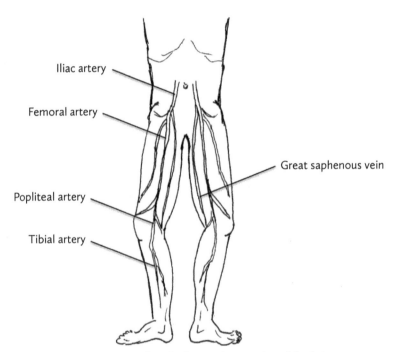

Diagram 11. Femoral and other major arteries of the legs

Location: Find the pulse of the femoral artery with your fingers or thumbs. It is slightly below the inguinal ligament in the crease between the leg and the pubic bone.

Technique: Compress with the heels of the palms and *hold steady* over the femoral artery

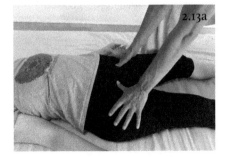

for 40–50 seconds and no more than 60 seconds.

Let go and brush down the legs with your hands "guiding" the flow of blood and energy downward.

Transition: to **Tripod.** From Lunge, step down and place your knees on the outside of the client's ankles.

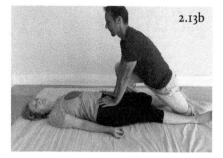

2.13b

Step 14. Palm press shin muscles

Push the client's ankles into internal hip rotation. Lock them in position with your knees.

Palm press into the anterior tibialis right along the edge of the tibia. Push the muscle "off" the bone.

Rock in to press in, rock out to release.

Go up and down 2 times.

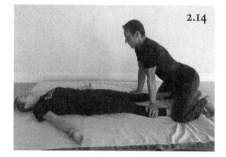

2.14

Supine—Single Leg Sequence

Step 15. Single leg traction

Grasp over the client's foot.

Squeeze the foot between your hands and thumbs and pull back.

Lean back with your body weight.

Rock back to pull, rock forward to release. Repeat 4–5 times.

A. Central hand hold.

B. Medial arch hold.

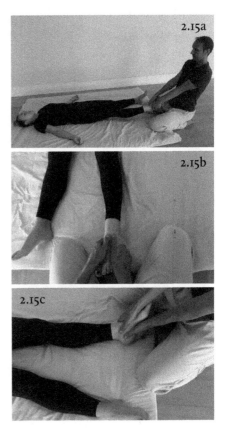

Step 16. Ankle rotations

Grasp over the client's toes and cup their heel.

Rotate the ankle 4–5 times each way.

Step 17. Ankle point circles (ST41)

This is a Wind Gate point, and also Point 41 on the Stomach meridian in the Chinese Meridian system.

Thumb circle into the ankle point.

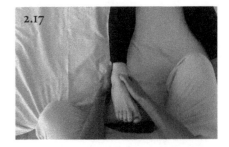

Do not be afraid to dig in to clear its energy. If the point is crunchy or tender, the energy has a blockage.

Step 18. Top of foot lines

There are 9 lines:

- 4 in the interosseus membranes between the metatarsals

- 5 on the tendons running out to each toe tip (**Diagram 12**).

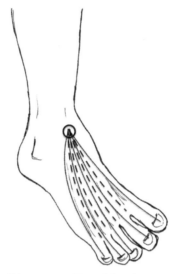

Diagram 12. Top of foot lines

Thumb circle from the ankle point down over the first 4 lines (between the metatarsals).

Thumb circle from the ankle point down to each toe-tip.

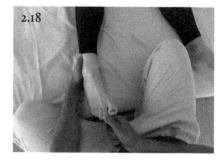

Squeeze gently at the toe-tip and quickly pull up to make a "popping" sound.

Hold the client's heel with the other hand. Switch hands as needed.

Step 19. Ankle point circles

Finger press and circle into the medial and lateral ankle points. Find dips and depressions around the malleoli.

If a point is tender or crunchy, there may be a blockage of energy or scar tissue.

Alternate technique: Hold a point and rotate the foot.

Cross-fiber friction medial and lateral ankle ligaments.

Transition (optional): Tripod to One-Leg-Out.

A. Inside leg straight, outside leg bent—rest the client's ankle on your inside leg.

B. Inside leg bent, outside leg straight—rest the client's ankle on your knee.

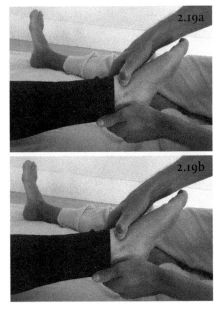

Step 20. Leg traction with ankle rotation

Place the client's foot and ankle over your knee or thigh, depending on the position (see above). Position their foot in front of your abdomen.

A. External rotation. Grasp over the client's foot close to the ankle joint with your outside hand and cup their heel with your inside hand.

Lean back with your body weight to traction the client's leg.

Twist their ankle into internal rotation 5 times, changing hand positions as follows: 1–2–3–2–1.

Hand positions: (1) low at ankle joint; (2) at mid-foot; (3) high at toe joints.

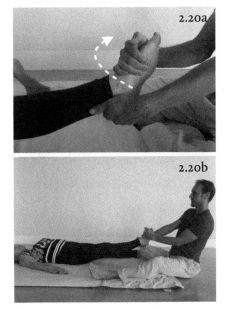

B. Internal rotation. Change hands—grasp over the client's foot with your inside hand, placing your thumb on the bottom of their foot. Cup the client's heel with your outside hand.

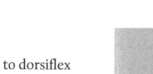

Perform leg traction as above: 1–2–3–2–1.

Step 21. Ankle wave push and pull

Hold the client's heel with your inside hand. Grasp over their toes with your outside hand.

Lift their foot up.

Press into the ball of the foot to dorsiflex their ankle.

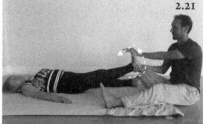

Keep it in dorsiflexion and lower the foot down.

Pull back on the foot or traction leg.

Lift the foot and repeat 5 times at the pace of 1 circle per second.

CLINICAL FOCUS #1: PLANTAR FASCIITIS

Plantar fasciitis is the inflammation of the fascia on the bottom of the foot due to strain and micro-tears. If the tissues are short, tight, and/or weak, and put under a lot of stress, they may get torn off of the attachments at the calcaneus (the heel bone) or along their length, usually close to the heel. Ouch! Weak and tight tissues are more susceptible to injury.

How does it happen? Say you decide to go hike or run 10 miles without gradual buildup of strength for that distance, or if you have to stand for three hours in poorly-fitting shoes. That's when plantar fasciitis may develop.

Neuromuscular Therapy (NMT) is an effective way of removing the scarring and treating plantar fasciitis.

Plantar fascia treatment

Rest the client's heel in your lap.

Push on the toes and/or the ball of the foot to gently stretch the plantar fascia.

Use your thumbs, fingers, and knuckles.

Begin with light cross-fiber friction along the Sen lines and fascial lines (refer to **Diagram 8**).

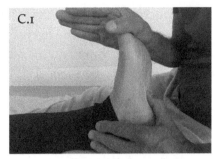

Look for *taut bands*, thin and thick, and for sensitive "hot" spots within those bands—this is usually where the tear (and scar tissue) is.

Once on a sensitive area, *strip it gently* (cross-fiber) at multiple angles, diagonal and perpendicular to the fibers. Cover the entire area in multiple strips.

If deeper pressure can be tolerated, perform the "pin and stretch" technique: thumb press and hold a hot spot, then push–release on the ball of the foot several times. Reposition to different spots and repeat.

Apply cooling gel or lotion at the end to "make nice."

Transition: One-Leg-Out. Reach over, bend the client's knee, and plant their foot down.

Scoot in and lock their shin with your ankle.

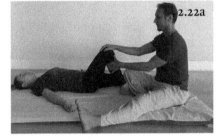

Step 22. Lower leg outside lines

See **Diagram 13** of outside leg lines and **Diagram 14** of the related muscles.

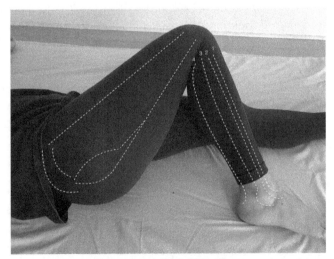

Diagram 13. Lateral leg lines

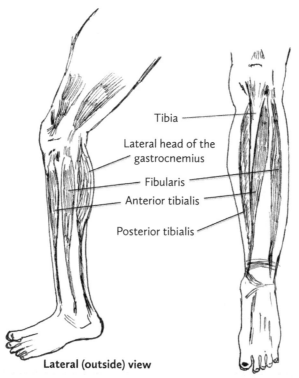

Tibia

Lateral head of the gastrocnemius

Fibularis

Anterior tibialis

Posterior tibialis

Lateral (outside) view

Diagram 14. Lower leg muscles

Line 1: Between the **tibia** and **anterior tibialis**, right next to the tibia.

Start right below the knee.

This point relates to **ST36** (see **Diagram 3** and **Table 1**) and is an immune system booster.

Thumb press 8–10 times into this point.

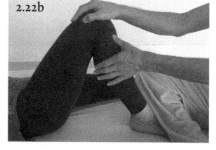

Then, move down 1 inch and perform 3 thumb presses in place—pluck the tissue away from the tibia.

Move down 1 inch at a time: 1–2–3 move down, 1–2–3 move down, and so on.

Line 2: In the myofascial compartment between the **anterior tibialis** and **fibularis** muscles.

Same technique as above. Thumb press 3 times and move down.

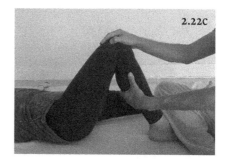

Line 3: On the **fibularis** muscle bundle.

Start just below the head of the fibula.

Twang over the ropey **fibularis** with your thumb or curved fingers, like plucking a string.

Line 4: This is the *posterior* outside line that runs over the lateral head of the **gastrocnemius**.

Hook your fingers and strum across or finger circle: 1–2–3 and move down.

It may be ropey—"strum the string."

Step 23. Hook fingers on calf

Hook your fingers on the center of the calf and pull back, "raking" out from the midline.

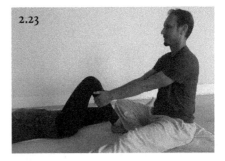

2.23

Muscles: Gastrocnemius and soleus.

Keep your arms straight and lean your body back.

"Make nice"—roll the calf between your palms. Soft fist-pound the calf gently.

CLINICAL FOCUS #2: ACHILLES TENDINITIS

The calves include the deeper-lying thicker **soleus**, and the more superficial double-headed **gastrocnemius** (**Diagram 15**). Both of these muscles merge into the **Achilles** tendon.

When these muscles get tight due to lack of exercise, lack of stretching, or too much exercise, the Achilles tendon gets tight, too. The Achilles tendon, as all other tendons in the body, is not elastic, meaning that it is a set length, incapable of being stretched beyond its length. To stretch a tendon is to tear it. Hence, the only way to gain some relief in the Achilles tendon from any tightness is to stretch its attaching muscles—the calves.

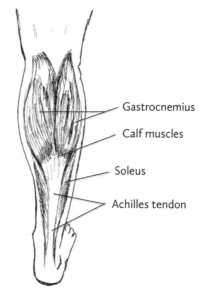

Diagram 15. Calf muscles

If the calves are not stretched and relaxed over time, the tension they exert on the tendon may cause tears and inflammation. This condition is generally known as Achilles tendinitis. You may see redness and an almond-sized bulge at the site of the injury and feel the bulge with your fingers. This bulge is the scar tissue forming around the tear. It is best prevented rather than treated.

To prevent it, advise your clients to stretch their calves on a regular basis and to strengthen the calves and Achilles tendon by performing calf raises and eccentric heel drops (see **Article 1** in the Appendix).

To treat tendonitis, focus on smoothing out the tissues and removing the scarring with light transverse cross-fiber friction, as explained below.

Technique: Perform Steps 22 and **23** above, to loosen the calves.

Stabilize the client's knee with one hand. Hook and strum your fingers across the musculotendinous junction where the **gastrocnemius** and **soleus** join together to form the Achilles tendon.

Strum across in multiple cross-fiber strokes down to the heel, beginning with the most lateral line of fibers moving across medially.

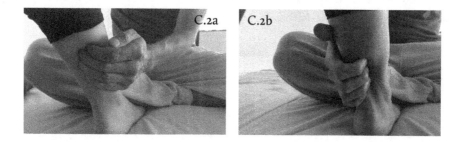

If the tear has formed a scar (an almond-shaped bulge), gently roll it between your thumb and fingers and "milk" it at different angles.

It helps tremendously to isolate the exact pinpoint of the tear. Apply cooling gel or lotion and cross-fiber friction on and through that pinpoint spot.

Caution: Do not spend more than 10 minutes on the area. Return to it if needed from a different position (for example, in prone).

CLINICAL FOCUS #3: KNEE JOINT AND LIGAMENTS

For pain inside the knee joint, that is, meniscus (cartilage) or anterior cruciate ligament (ACL), there is not much we can do as massage therapists and body-workers but soothe and relax the surrounding tissues. This is a good case of sending your client to a specialist like an orthopedic doctor. We can, however, check for ACL tears or instability and cross-fiber friction or treat exterior ligaments, as in the techniques below.

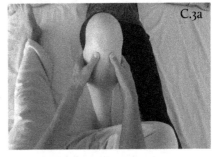
C.3a

ACL test: Hook your fingers at the top of the calves.

Pull back and watch the client's knee.

If their knee pulls out visibly like a sliding drawer (i.e., the tibia shifts forward from under the femur), it is likely that the ACL has been torn, or loosened, as it is not holding the tibia in place. This looseness creates knee joint insta-bility and makes the knee more prone to injury. Clients must strengthen their knee-attaching muscles to compensate for that instability (quads, adductors, hamstrings).

Knee ligament treatment

When the pain or scar tissue is in and around the patellar ligament (patellar tendinitis), medial or lateral collateral ligaments (MCL and LCL tears), and/or meniscus (medial and lateral injuries or tears), we can focus to break up and reduce the scar tissue with cross-fiber friction techniques (**Diagram 16**).

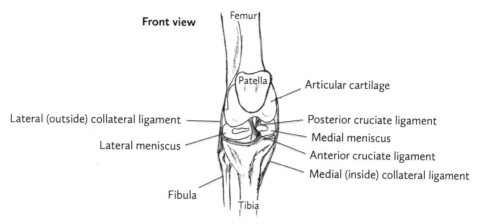

Front view

Femur

Patella

Articular cartilage

Lateral (outside) collateral ligament

Posterior cruciate ligament

Lateral meniscus

Medial meniscus

Anterior cruciate ligament

Medial (inside) collateral ligament

Fibula

Tibia

Diagram 16. Anterior knee bones and ligaments

Cross-fiber friction over the patellar ligament at different transverse angles.

Use your thumb and fingers.

Cross-fiber friction around the patella, focusing on the medial and lateral aspects.

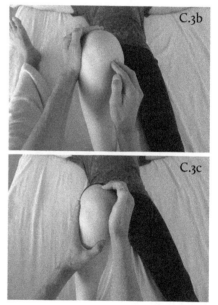

C.3b

Cross-fiber friction above the patella, at the musculotendinous tissues of the quads.

Cross-fiber friction gently into:

- MCL between the tibia and the femur.

- LCL between the fibula, tibia, and the femur.

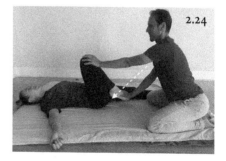

C.3c

Transition: One-Leg-Out to **Lunge.** Lean on to your inside arm. With your outside hand, push the client's knee up so that their foot lifts off the floor.

Step 24. Knee flexion 1–2–3

Press over the client's toes—"heel to butt."

Mild–medium–deep.

Hold on "deep" for 3 seconds.

Repeat 2 times.

Caution: Be careful not to push too hard as many people's knees have a limited ROM.

2.24

Step 25. Hip flexion 1–2–3

Hold the client's knee and heel. Press their knee to same-side shoulder. Repeat several times.

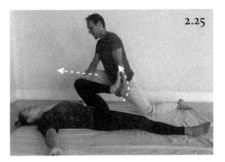

2.25

Caution: Do not press the client's knee to the opposite shoulder! This may impinge their inguinal ligament.

Cup the client's heel and press your forearm over their foot into dorsiflexion.

Step up higher to provide a deeper flexion for their ankle. And rock! 1–2–3.

Hold for 4–5 seconds at the deepest point.

Application: Improves hip joint mobility and helps relieve lower back tension.

Transition (optional): Switch legs. **Lunge** to **Lunge** or **Archer**. Bring one knee down, the other knee up. This will help you rest your inside elbow on your inside knee.

Step 26. Hip internal and external rotation check

Hold the client's heel with your inside hand and guide their knee with your outside hand.

Turn their hip into external and internal rotation several times. (External rotation is shown in Photo 2.26a and internal rotation in Photo 2.26b.) Check the maximum comfortable ROM.

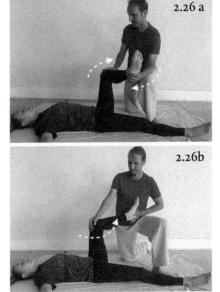

2.26 a

2.26b

Step 27. Hip circles

Guide the client's leg in outward circles—press toward the shoulder and go outward.

Start with small circles. Progress to wider circles and to the edge of their ROM.

Circle each way 4–5 times.

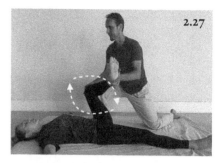

2.27

Step 28. Hip joint traction

Hook your upper forearm under the client's knee.

Pull to traction their leg outward.

Transition: Tripod in place.

Add circles. Pull–release—bounce it!

Variation: Downward traction. Bring the client's foot down and lock it down with your hand.

Pull–release downward 4–5 times.

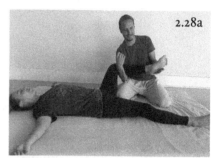

2.28a

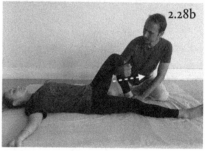

2.28b

Step 29. "Arm cracker"

Pinch your forearm between the client's calf and hamstring by pressing the client's foot down (heel to butt).

Roll your forearm in place.

Release, reposition, repeat 4–5 times.

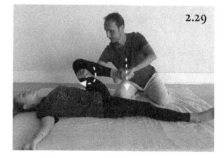

2.29

Step 30. The number 4

(*For flexible clients.*)

Transition: pivot in **Tripod** to face the client.

Place the client's ankle over their opposite thigh. Support their knee (if not touching the floor) with your knee in **Tripod**.

Technique: Palm press the client's thigh up and down 2–3 times. Start with very light pressure and progress to deeper pressure.

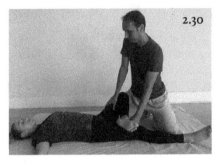

2.30

Step 31. Tree Pose

A. Place the client's foot at their inner thigh. Support their leg with your outside knee if needed. Lock their ankle with your inside knee.

Rock in and out to palm press the thigh and calf 2–3 times, up and down.

Muscles: Adductors, vastus medialis, calves.

B. Butterfly palm press. Bring the heels of your palms together.

C. Palm walk opposite thighs. Rock side to side. Palm press gently and keep your knee under the client's leg, especially if it does not touch the ground.

D. Forearm press.

Transition: down to **Low Tripod.**

Use your outside elbow for vastus medialis/ quads.

Use your inside elbow for the adductor muscles.

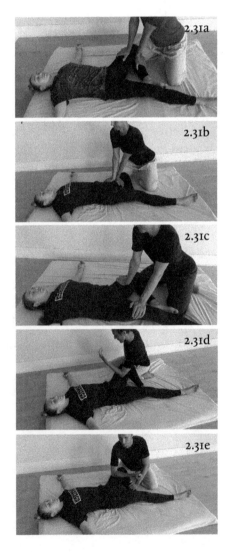

2.31a

2.31b

2.31c

2.31d

2.31e

Step 32. Hip adduction palm press

From **Tree Pose**, slide the client's leg out, lift their knee and press it into adduction. Bring your knee at their ankle to prevent the leg from straightening.

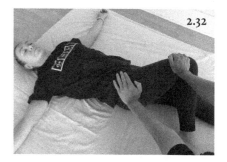

Palm press along **ITB** and from hip to knee. Rock palm to palm.

Palm circle around the greater trochanter.

Step 33. Lateral leg lines

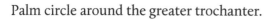

Line 1 (continuous with lower leg line 1): on the anterior lateral aspect of the femur; roughly between the vastus lateralis and ITB, and between the anterior gluteus medius and **tensor fasciae latae (Diagram 17)**.

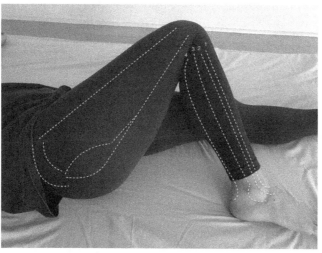

Diagram 17. Lateral leg lines

Thumb-chasing-thumb: Start at the top of the line. Point thumbs at each other. The technique is "press down and pull." The top thumb catches up to the lower thumb in roughly 1-inch segments.

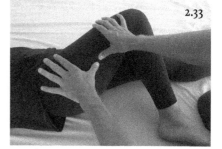

Line 2 (continuous with lower leg line 3): Centerline of ITB and gluteus medius.

Line 3 (continuous with lower leg line 4 or posterior lateral line): On the posterior lateral aspect of the femur, roughly between the ITB and biceps femoris, and along the posterior edge of the greater trochanter.

Step 34. Outside leg palm press

Straighten the client's leg. Palm press from ankle to hip over all lines.

Keep your arms straight. Rock your body side to side.

Variation: Lateral leg lines. Perform this technique instead of Step 33, as needed.

Thumb-chasing-thumb: Skip line 3 if hard to access.

Transition: Tripod to **One-Leg-Out.** Lift the client's heel. Lean on your inside arm and sit under the client's mid-calf, facing away from their head.

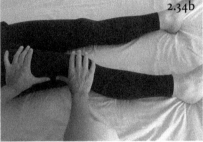

Step 35. Finger hook on foot

Hook your fingers and lean back. Rock back several times.

Finger walk up or down over the client's plantar fascia.

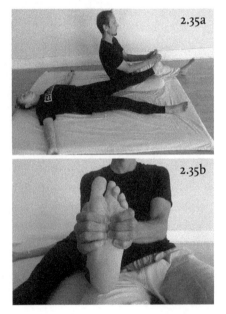

Step 36. Squeeze top of foot

Glide thumbs over the top of the foot, slowly, without "skin burn."

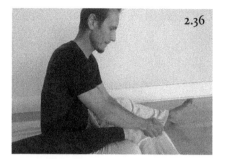

2.36

Step 37. Ankle dorsiflexion with Achilles tendon squeeze

Use your outside hand to grasp over the client's foot and cup their heel. Pull their ankle into dorsiflexion.

Squeeze the Achilles tendon between your thumb and fingers while "cranking" the ankle (dorsiflexing).

"Make nice" with soft fist-pound over the calf, 8–10 times.

Press over the client's toes and soft fist-pound the bottom of the foot.

Transition C: One-Leg-Out to **Lunge.**

2.37a

2.37b

Step 38. Straight leg test with ankle lock

Rest the client's calf over your thigh. Cup over their heel.

Rock from side to side, pulling the client's ankle into dorsiflexion, and palm press down their thigh, 1–2–3–2–1.

This move is known as the straight leg raise (SLR) test to check for sciatica.

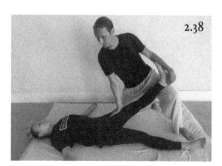

2.38

As needed, continue with **Clinical focus #12** on **sciatica.**

Step 39. Crossover leg stretch

Transition: Step over the client's other leg.

Cup the client's heel and rest their ankle over your thigh.

A. Gentle stretch (for clients with limited hip ROM, especially in adduction, as in after a hip replacement surgery). Palm press down lTB, 1–2–3–2–1.

Palm circle at the greater trochanter.

Muscles/tissues: ITB, vastus lateralis, gluteus medius, tensor fascia latae.

B. Medium stretch. Step farther out across. Bring your knee closer.

Slide your elbow onto your knee to extend the stretch. Keep a hold of the client's heel.

Palm press and circle as above.

"Pin and stretch"—hold down tissue at the hip and lower the client's leg past your knee, 4–5 times.

C. Deep stretch. Lower the client's leg all the way to the floor. Make sure it's at close to 90 degrees across. Lock their leg with your ankle.

Palm press as above.

Elbow press and roll the muscles around the greater trochanter.

"Make nice"—soft fist-pound and chop-chop lTB and around the greater trochanter.

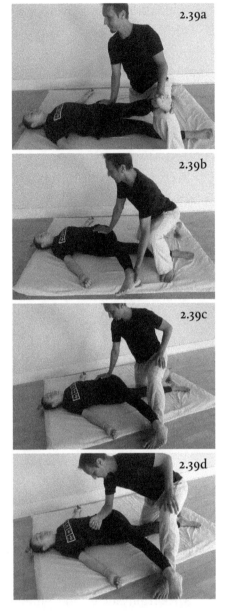

2.39a

2.39b

2.39c

2.39d

Step 40. Hip abduction stretch

Transition: Lunge to Archer.

Step back over the client's leg.

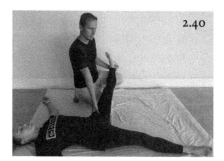

2.40

Hold the client's heel. Scoot back away from the client, taking their leg out into abduction.

Pull their leg into the abduction stretch: 1–2–3, mild–medium–deep.

Hold on "deep" for 8–10 seconds to let them "enjoy" the stretch.

Palm press and/or thumb press at their hip flexor muscles.

Hook the client's ankle over your knee. Hold for 8–10 seconds.

Transition: to Tripod.

Step 41. Calf press and roll

Rest the client's calf over your lower thigh. Hold under their heel.

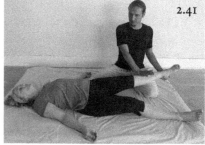

2.41

Rock your body forward and back, and simultaneously palm press into the **anterior tibialis**.

Press and roll their calf over your thigh.

Lift the client's leg by the heel to reposition your lower leg to address the full length of their calf muscles.

Step 42. Thigh press and roll

Slide your upper knee under the client's thigh.

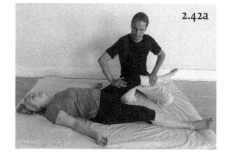

2.42a

Start with palm press and roll over the **quads**.

Continue with elbow or forearm press and roll.

Muscles: Releases the quadriceps, especially the vastus lateralis and rectus femoris, and the tensor fascia latae.

Additional elbow/forearm techniques:

A. "Hook in and sink" compressions. With the elbow, target the **tensor fascia latae** and anterior **gluteus medius**.

B. Cross-fiber compressions from the **rectus femoris** tendon and **tensor fascia latae** down to the distal **quadriceps** attachments on the femur.

C. With the forearm, press into the **ITB** and roll over the **quads**.

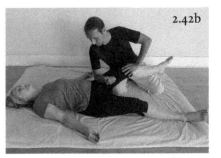

2.42b

Step 43. Anterior tibialis release

A. Knee press. This is a deeper technique following previous softer techniques to relax the **anterior tibialis**.

Rotate the client's leg medially and hold on to their foot.

Place your knee (either one) directly on their **anterior tibialis**.

Sink gently and slowly, then rock your knee up or down and side-to-side in place.

Move along the tibia.

Repeat 2 times.

B. Double-thumb press. This is a more specific targeted technique.

Thumb-over-thumb press and cross-fiber friction along the **anterior tibialis** and **fibularis**.

Alternate with "A" as needed.

C. Palm press with ankle lock. Lock the client's foot with your lower knee.

Rock side to side to palm press and "crank" the client's ankle into dorsiflexion.

Transition: Hero.

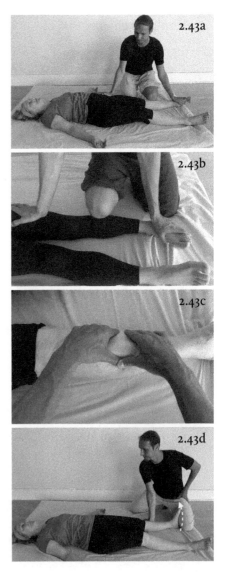

2.43a

2.43b

2.43c

2.43d

Step 44. Hamstrings release

Pick up the client's leg and sit facing their head. Hold their heel.

Lift the client's leg up to a comfortable resistance point.

Use your body weight—lean in and lock your elbow, to stretch their hamstrings.

Use your outside hand to keep the client's knee from bending.

A. Thumb press and stretch. Use your outside hand to "thumb pluck the strings" of the hamstrings.

Cross-fiber friction across the hamstrings, top to bottom.

Pick a line of tissue and follow it all the way down to the ischial tuberosity.

B. Thumb press with ankle over shoulder. Rest the client's ankle on your inside shoulder. Inch up closer if needed.

Thumb strum the strings side to side, pulling away from the midline. I call this "playing the cello."

C. Thumb press with foot rest (*for stiff or injured clients*). Rest the client's foot against your abdomen. Strum across their hamstrings.

Hold their knee up with your other hand.

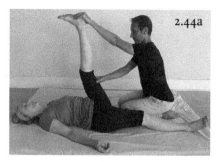

2.44a

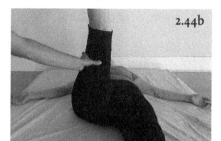

2.44b

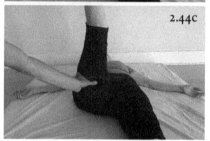

2.44c

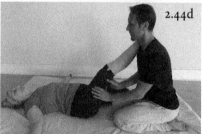

2.44d

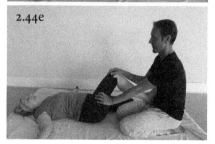

2.44e

Step 45. Quadriceps release

Keep the client's ankle on your inside shoulder.

Hook your fingers on the center line of the quads.

A. Finger walk and circle. Press and circle away from the midline. Strum over the ropey **rectus femoris**.

With your outside hand, finger circle (and strum across) the hip flexor muscle bundle.

B. Palm squeeze and traction. Interlace your fingers over the client's thigh.

Squeeze the thigh or quads between your palms and lean back.

Reposition your grasp and repeat. Low–middle–high. 1–2–3–2–1.

Rock back and forward to traction.

"Make nice"—quick roll the thigh between your palms. Soft fist-pound the quads.

Transition: to **Archer.** Curl your toes under. Lift your inside knee up.

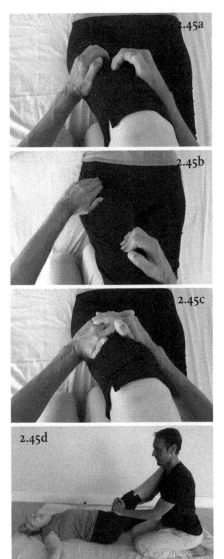

2.45a

2.45b

2.45c

2.45d

Step 46. Hamstrings knee press

A. Inside knee press. Hold the client's foot at the heel.

Hold over the client's knee with your outside hand.

Press your knee into the hamstrings as you pull the client's leg closer.

Press your knee by flexing your foot into the floor.

Go up and down 2–3 times.

"Pin and stretch"—press your knee near the hamstrings attachments and stretch the client's leg up.

Push at the heel.

Rock in and out. Reposition your knee 4–5 times.

Add a thumb press across the hamstrings.

B. Outside knee press. Switch knees.

Target the posterior lateral line, that is, the biceps femoris.

"Pin and stretch" on this line, as above.

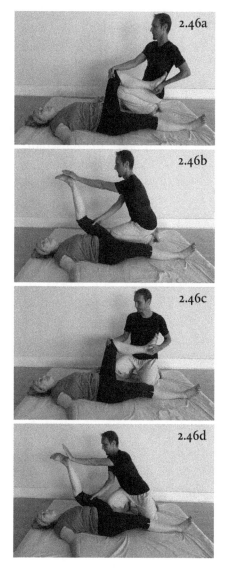

2.46a

2.46b

2.46c

2.46d

CLINICAL FOCUS #4: HAMSTRING TEARS AND HIGH HAMSTRING TENDINOPATHY

Hamstring pulls and tears are common among recreational and professional athletes. If the hamstrings are very tight and not warmed up properly before exercise, there is a higher chance of injury. Runners, cyclists, soccer players, lacrosse players, and other athletes experience hamstring pulls and tears on a regular basis. Often, an athlete may hear a "pop" in the back of their leg, followed by tenderness or pain, a pulling sensation, and a black-and-blue mark.

It is important to let these tears heal and not stretch the healing tissue.

Otherwise, it can be re-torn and become even more damaged. When healing tissues are re-injured over and over again, an internal scar (adhesion) is formed at the site of the injury, causing tightness and a restricted range of movement.

While it is helpful to stretch the hamstrings when they are healthy (not torn), it is contraindicated to stretch these muscles during the healing phase. Instead, a strengthening routine and regular Neuromuscular Therapy (NMT) will accelerate the healing process.

High hamstring tendinopathy is a chronic re-tearing and scarring of the hamstrings at the musculotendinous junction (**Diagram 18**). This is where the three hamstrings converge into one single tendon and is the most common site of chronic injury. Hence the name, tendinopathy.

This re-tearing usually occurs due to weak gluteals, as well as short and weak hamstrings, and a lack of stretching and strengthening of the hamstrings.

High hamstring tendinopathy is a persistent condition that may take several months or even a year to resolve. Strengthening the hamstrings and the glutes is essential in the process of healing. NMT will also help to break up adhesions and restore normal function.

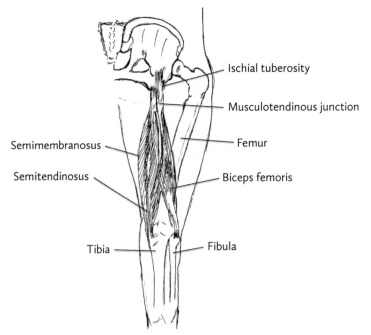

Diagram 18. Hamstrings – posterior leg view

The hamstrings protocol

1. Perform **Step 44** above. Look for adhesions and cross-fiber friction at the site of injury at diagonal angles. Use your thumbs or knuckles to be

muscle-fiber specific. Switch your hands as needed to give your thumbs a rest.

2. Add "pin and stretch" compressions, pushing the client's leg up at the heel.

3. Perform **Step 46**.

4. Alternate between **Steps 44** and **46** if necessary.

5. Continue to **prone** with **Step 98** ("palm walk upper legs" up the hamstrings) and **Step 99** ("medial upper legs lines" on the upper legs).

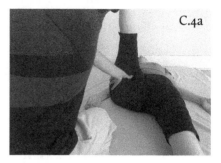

6. Thumb walk right on the hamstrings (same technique as #5). Look for tight strips of tissue and focus your cross-fiber friction at those stripped sites.

7. In **prone**, lift the client's opposite ankle and step to **Lunge** over their straight leg.

8. With your upper hand, thumb press across the hamstrings. Look for adhesions and cross-fiber friction to remove scar tissue.

9. Add the "pin and stretch" technique. Bring the client's ankle down (extend the knee) while pinning down at a specific spot on the hamstrings.

10. Change spots and repeat multiple times.

11. Additionally, knuckle roll up the hamstrings while extending the knee.

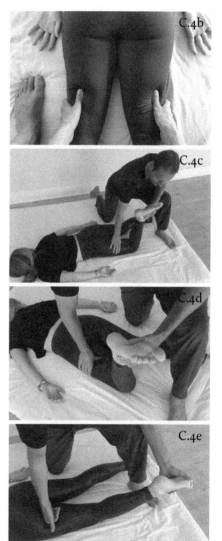

Step 47. Foot press in hamstring stretch

(For clients of a similar size to the therapist!)

Transition: Tai Chi stance. Stand up with feet apart at walking stance.

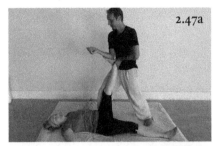

Rest the client's foot against your abdomen.

Lock the client's knee from the side with your front leg.

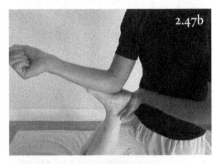

Cup the client's foot with your inside hand and elbow roll into their foot.

Switch hands as needed.

Transition: Lunge down (with outside leg).

Step 48. Pigeon Pose

Hold the client's heel and knee.

A. Rock 1–2–3, light–medium–deep.

Press and hold on "deep."

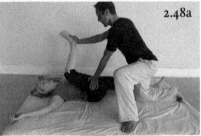

B. Transition to Archer Pose, with your inside knee up.

Press your knee gently over the client's opposite thigh.

Repeat the technique from "A."

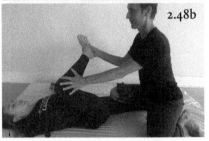

Transition: Lunge (outside leg).

Step 49. Hip flexion with thigh palm press

Place the client's foot at your hip crease. Make sure to lock their heel in front of your anterior iliac crest.

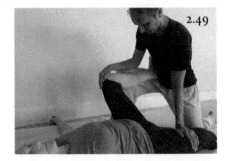

Rock forward and back.

Guide the client's knee to their shoulder, and palm press their opposite thigh, 1–2–3–2–1.

Step 50. Adductor palm press

Step your front foot out. Keep the client's foot in front of your hip. Hold their knee.

Palm press their adductors.

Rock in and out, 1–2–3–2–1.

Repeat 2–3 times.

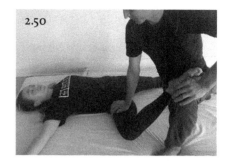

Step 51. Adductor stretch

Step your foot out. Straighten the client's leg slowly to avoid overstretching.

Check in with the client.

Lock their leg with your ankle.

Return to previous position: Bring the client's foot into the front of your hip.

Gently palm press the adductors (this technique does not require deep pressure).

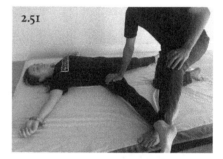

Step 52. Adductors elbow press

Transition B: Lunge to **One-Leg-Out.** Keep the client's foot in your hip. Lean on your inside arm and slide your knee under the client's thigh.

Two options for the client's foot placement: Lock their foot on your thigh (Photo 2.52) or place their foot over your thigh.

Techniques: Forearm or elbow press and roll. Use your inside arm.

Rock and press along the length of their adductors.

Hold deeper compressions as needed.

Cross-fiber friction as needed.

Transition: Pivot away from the client—sit facing away from them.

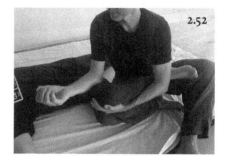

Step 53. Quadriceps elbow press

Use your inside elbow or forearm.

Supinate: Press your elbow or forearm with your palm facing down, then turn your palm up.

Roll over the quads, up or down, 2–3 times.

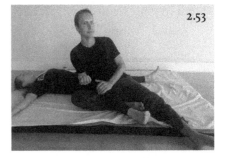

2.53

Step 54. Paddleboat, aka bicycle

Transition from Step 53: Turn toward the client. Keep the client's knee out at 90 degrees.

Place your feet on the client's hamstrings.

Hold under their ankle.

Place your inside hand on the client's other ankle (if the client's legs are long, grasp over their knee).

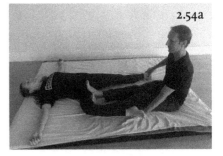

2.54a

Technique: Paddle and rock your body forward and back.

Press your outside foot in (the foot at the client's knee) and lean forward.

Press your inside foot in, rock back, and pull on the client's legs.

Use your feet, heels, or balls of the feet when pressing into the hamstrings.

Walk along the length of the hamstrings 4–5 times.

Where to sit: The right spot is where you can straighten your outside leg and bring the client's knee out to a minimum of 90 degrees (right angle). If their knee is bent at less than 90 degrees, you are sitting too low, or too far away from them.

Variation: "Foot knife"—keep your outside knee slightly bent and hook the client's foot on the inside of your knee. Lean back on your arms.

Use your inside foot: Press deep and turn your foot on its lateral edge and hold for 6–8 seconds.

Roll up to release.

Repeat 4–5 times along the length of the hamstrings.

While holding deep compressions, wiggle your stationary foot (optional).

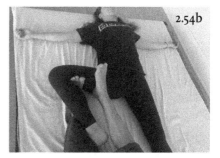

Step 55. Thigh compression

Sit closer to the client. Keep your knees bent.

Hook the client's foot over your knees.

Grasp your hands over their thigh and pull back.

Palm walk across their thigh while simultaneously foot pressing the thigh.

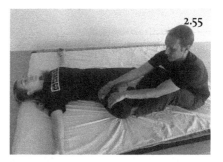

Step 56. Adductor stretch and heel press

Stretch the client's leg out to a comfortable point of resistance.

Curl your toes back and place *their heel* (not the Achilles tendon) over your toes, between your big toe and second toe.

If the stretch is too gentle, their heel will fall off your foot.

Find a stretch that is taut or tight enough so their heel rests over your toes by itself.

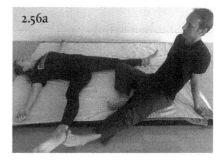

After letting the client enjoy the stretch for 10–15 seconds, place your heel on the **adductors**.

Rest your heel without adding any extra pressure or weight.

This can be very sensitive! Even a gentle touch (with your heel) may be too much.

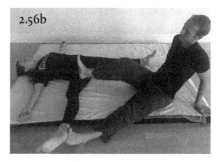

Reposition to different spots on the adductors.

Note: Stay away from the knee. Keep close to the groin.

Step 57. Hamstrings foot press, and/or leg lift transition

Use your outside foot and push it into the client's hamstrings. Grasp the client's ankle and pull.

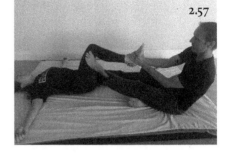

2.57

With this counter-tension, lift their leg up to 90 degrees.

Turn your foot out so your toes point out.

Foot press into the hamstrings and lean back.

Step 58. Leg extension, aka "123 automatic"

Drop your heel (outside leg) down and place your foot against the client's leg.

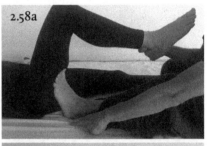

2.58a

Make sure your foot is in the centerline of the hamstrings. Curl your toes back. Keep your foot planted in place.

Holding on to the client's ankle, lean back and pull their leg with you.

Lean back as far as comfortable.

Traction the leg for 3–4 seconds.

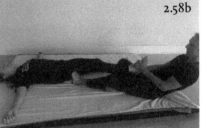

2.58b

Ischial tuberosity press: Lift and push the client's knee toward their chest. As their leg goes up, your foot will naturally gain a deeper (higher) placement on the hamstrings. Do not move your foot! Keep it planted in place.

Lean back again and take the leg with you.

Repeat several times until the ball of your foot is at the client's ischial tuberosity.

Rock your foot back and forth. Wiggle your foot or toes side to side.

To finish, lift the client's leg and bring your foot out.

Step 59. Quadriceps finger walk

Plant the client's foot and slide it closer to their buttock. Lock their ankle with your inside leg.

Hook your fingers on the midline of the quads.

Walk your fingers up and down, pulling away from the midline.

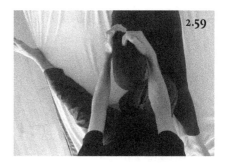

Step 60. Squeeze thigh and traction hip

Keep the client's ankle locked, as above.

Interlace your fingers over their thigh and lean back with straight arms.

Change your hand placement with every pull: high–middle–low, as in 1–2–3–2–1.

Special transition: Push the client's knee up with your outside hand and dangle their foot to "unlock" the hip.

Drop their foot out, away from the midline, into internal hip rotation.

From here, continue with **Transition B**, then into **Archer**.

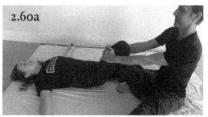

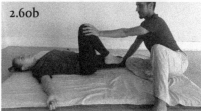

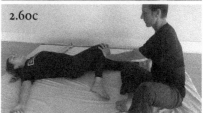

Step 61. Internal hip rotation press

Place your knee anywhere along the **ITB**. Support the client's knee with your hand if needed.

Knee press gently along the ITB, rocking in and out.

Avoid the greater trochanter.

Knee press into the **gluteus medius**.

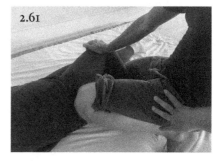

CLINICAL FOCUS #5: THE GLUTEUS MEDIUS

The gluteus medius is one of the most important muscles for balance and stability (**Diagram 19**). Even before the "core" muscles react, the gluteus medius kicks in every time we take a step. Its job is to stabilize the femur in its socket, as well as to perform internal and external hip rotation.

The gluteus medius gets tight and overworked and causes a slew of common conditions and imbalances, which are often missed or misunderstood, such as ITB syndrome and runner's knee and even high hamstring tendinopathy. (See **Article 2** in the Appendix for more information on the **ITB** and the **gluteus medius.**)

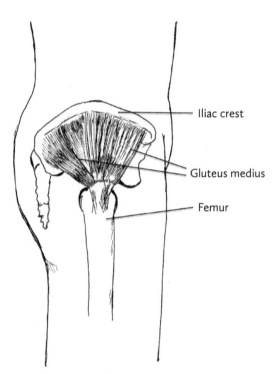

Iliac crest

Gluteus medius

Femur

Diagram 19. The Gluteus Medius

We have already performed a variety of techniques that help stretch and treat the gluteus medius. The following position is another option. Additionally, **Step 65** below is a great technique to address the gluteus medius.

Positioning: If comfortable for the client, keep their leg in internal rotation, as in **Step 61**.

Hand-over-hand cross-fiber friction at the **anterior gluteus medius**, and along the superior iliac crest. Or thumb press and cross-fiber friction.

If the client's internal hip rotation is limited, straighten their leg and prop their hip up with your knee under the gluteus medius.

Friction up and down and side to side to unstick or separate the fibers between the **tensor fascia latae** and **anterior gluteus medius**.

Move from anterior to posterior in horizontal strips, searching for sensitive areas and TPs.

Compress those sensitive nodules (TPs) and hold for 8–10 seconds. Repeat as needed.

"Make nice" by grasping lightly and palm circling around the hip.

Transition: Step to **Lunge** on the same side.

Step 62: Lumbar traction

Hook your fingers on the posterior iliac crest (at the **quadratus lumborum**) and pull downward.

Pull–release 4–5 times.

Application: Relieves lower back tension.

Caution: Do not lift the client's knee straight up from this position. It may damage their hip labrum. To transition back into the straight-leg position, push the client's heel and knee inward first, in a circular motion, to bring their leg into the hip outward-circling move.

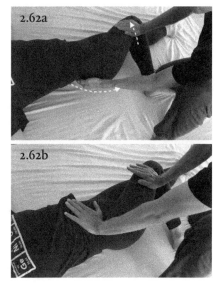

Variation: Palm press the obliques. Palm press on the side of the abdomen and the knee.

Rock side to side.

Palm press and hold the **obliques** to melt deeper toward the psoas.

A: Hook fingers on the posterior iliac crest.

B: Palm press the obliques.

Alternate between "A" and "B."

Step 63. Lower back reset

Transition: Step across the client's hips in **Lunge**.

Scoop under their lower ribs. Use your body weight—lean back and lift the client's lower back.

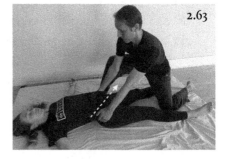
2.63

Repeat 3–4 times.

This technique resets the alignment of the lumbar spine after deep and detailed body-work on one side.

You may also perform this technique *after* any of the following:

- Deep glute knee press (**Step 64**).
- Iliopsoas release (**Clinical focus #6**).
- ITB and gluteus medius release and quadratus lumborum foot press (**Steps 65** and **66**).
- Hip abduction (**Step 67**).

Optional side switch: Move down to the client's foot. Traction their leg, as in **Step 68**, and let it go.

Begin the sequence from the top on the other side.

This switch can be performed now, or after any of the following five techniques: **Step 64**, the **psoas release**, and **Steps 65, 66**, and **67**.

Step 64. Deep glute knee press

Transition: to **Tripod**.

Use your upper knee. Hold the client's knee and heel.

Push their leg across into a semi-side lying position to lift their hip off the ground.

Slide your knee under, all the way to the sacrum. Your knee should cover the entire **gluteus maximus** area.

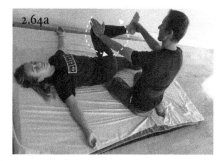

Pull the client back over your knee, letting their own weight compress into your knee.

Keep a hold on their knee and heel.

Circle and explore their hip ROM—with their foot up, then with their foot down.

Variation: Spiral position.

Transition: Spiral.

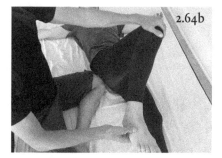

Push the client's leg across as in the previous move, and sit with your *upper knee* under the gluteus maximus.

This position provides a slightly deeper angle in the compressions.

Variation: Leg drape. Lean back on your arms and drape your free leg over the client's knee.

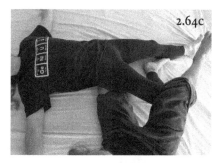

Use only the weight of your leg.

Caution: Do not press your leg down. This move requires a highly mobile hip joint in clients and may damage the hip joint if pressed down too quickly or too deeply.

CLINICAL FOCUS #6: THE ILIOPSOAS

The iliopsoas is one of the deepest and most important muscles in the body. Its main action is hip flexion. However, it assists other muscles with lumbar extension and overall spinal and postural stability.

It is the only hip flexor that crosses the pelvic region from top to bottom and originates at the lumbar spine (**Diagram 20**). Its unique position makes the iliopsoas perform this critical balancing and postural stability work. For example, standing on one leg and flexing the hip (raising the knee up) on one side helps your standing leg balance, prevents your pelvis from tilting forward, and keeps your back upright; on the other side it allows you to raise the knee higher than 90 degrees.

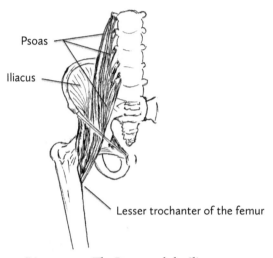

Psoas

Iliacus

Lesser trochanter of the femur

Diagram 20. The Psoas and the Iliacus

The iliopsoas is also a commonly missed and misdiagnosed cause of many conditions such as back pain, hip pain, and lumbar lordosis (deep curve in the lower back). Any time your client complains of lower back pain, always check and work on the iliopsoas.

The iliopsoas becomes chronically tight in active teenagers going through a growth spurt; athletes involved in repetitive hip flexion like running, cycling, soccer, and rowing; and inactive adults sitting in hip-flexed positions at their desks all day.

You may have seen young athletes, especially sprinters and hurdlers, develop a deep lumbar lordosis. As their bones grow long, their muscles are not able to catch up to the bone growth and stay short due to the high volume of exercise. These tight and short psoas muscle fibers exert tremendous pull on the lumbar spine, causing it to curve in, often resulting in muscle pulls, back pain, and other postural distortions.

Fortunately, the psoas is a thick muscle with many fibers. If some of its fibers are torn or pulled, others will compensate. In all of my practice, I have only seen one case of a total iliopsoas rupture. It was in a 17-year-old male lacrosse athlete. His psoas tore clean off its inferior attachment at the lesser trochanter when he twisted mid-run to hit a ball. Needless to say, it was a career-ending injury that caused years of pain and multiple surgeries on the psoas and the spine. When I met the athlete, he was 34 years old and still suffering from postural instability and pain.

Another example of a psoas-caused chronic pain condition was in a 60-year-old taxicab driver from Boston. His hip pain got so bad that he had a hard time getting out of his taxicab. He had to use his arms to lift his leg out of his seat. He told me he had been to doctors and physical therapists, and was given pain meds for his back pain and stretching exercises to relieve the back tension. No one told him about the psoas. Upon testing him, I could tell it was his chronically short iliopsoas that caused his discomfort and pain, probably from sitting for long periods of time in his taxicab. He had never heard of this muscle before.

I had to work in the side-lying position to get his abdomen out of the way to access his psoas. Even a gentle compression caused this man to start sweating and tearing up. After the first session, he was able to get up and walk without pain for the first time in months. He reported to me later that his issue resolved completely after our second treatment. I also encouraged him to stretch and strengthen his iliopsoas on a regular basis with quad stretches and leg lift exercises.

The iliopsoas release

Position: Tripod or **Hero.**

Optional: Prop up the client's knee and hip under your knee. This is my preferred position (Photos C.6b and C.6c).

ILIACUS
Hook your fingers over the iliac crest.

Let your fingers "melt" down the "ski slope" of the iliac crest into the iliacus.

Hold a steady compression for 8–10 seconds. Reposition and repeat 2–3 times.

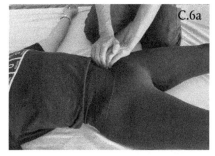

C.6a

PSOAS
Perform 3–4 hand-over-hand compressions.

Enter at the 45-degree angle off the edge of the **rectus abdominus**.

Follow the client's breath and melt down toward the lumbar vertebrae on their exhalation.

Upon reaching the muscle, hold for 10–15 seconds before releasing. If taut and ropey, cross-fiber friction during a steady deep compression.

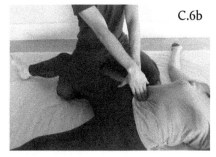

C.6b

Variation: Releasing the psoas with movement. This technique requires skill and good arm strength and is very effective—it allows therapists to access the psoas through multiple angles while the muscle is shortening and lengthening passively.

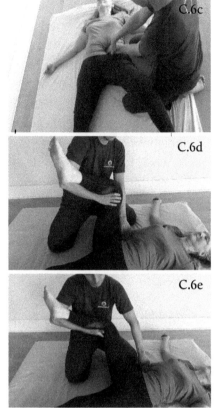

C.6c

C.6d

C.6e

Hold the client's lower leg underneath with your lower hand, gripping their leg under the knee (fingers inside, thumb outside).

As above, slowly melt your upper hand (finger pads) into the psoas at the 45-degree angle. Upon reaching the muscle fibers, rock your body side to side and in a circular way, moving the client's leg into extension, flexion, and hip rotation. Continue for 30–40 seconds. Direct your fingerpads toward the spine at different angles.

Bring the client's leg all the way down. Jostle and brush down the leg to "make nice."

Step 65. ITB and gluteus medius release

This is yet another effective way to release the gluteus medius (see **Clinical focus #5**).

Apply the cross-fiber and TP techniques using your heel and foot!

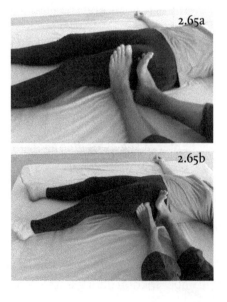

2.65a

2.65b

Sit back and place your feet on the client's ITB.

ITB technique: Press, turn, and catch up.

Press down gently with the upper foot.

Turn it on its lateral edge.

Press the bottom foot where the upper foot is lifted.

Repeat until reaching the greater trochanter.

Gluteus medius technique: Foot walk to roll the client's hip half way off the mat. Place your bottom foot all the way under the gluteus maximus (this is the support foot).

Heel press with your upper foot into the **gluteus medius**.

Compress and hold for 5–6 seconds.

Release and reposition.

Cross-fiber friction with your heel on the posterior, middle, and anterior fibers of the **gluteus medius** and **tensor fascia latae**.

Step 66. Quadratus lumborum foot press

Support the client's hip with your bottom foot (under the greater trochanter).

Turn your upper foot in (invert) and press the lateral edge of the foot into the "quadratus lumborum space"—between the iliac crest and lower ribs.

Aim toward the transverse processes.

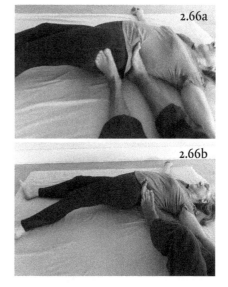

Hold for 6–8 seconds on each compression. Tell the client to breathe slowly.

For deeper compressions, let go of their greater trochanter—pull away your bottom foot, and let the client's weight roll back into your compression.

Application: Releases the quadratus lumborum, obliques, and transverse abdominis.

Variation: Double-foot press, for deeper compressions.

Step 67. Hip abduction with gluteus medius heel press

Hook your bottom toes under the client's ankle.

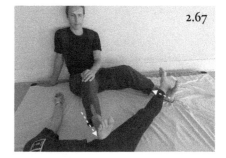

Set your upper heel into the client's gluteus medius. Traction the client's leg out to a *comfortable resistance* point.

Press (your heel) and pull (their leg).

Perform 6–8 compressions, changing your angle of pressure.

Step 68. Leg finish: palm press and roll and brush it out

Transition: to **Tripod.**

Bring the client's leg back into the straight position.

Palm press from foot to hip and roll the leg in/out.

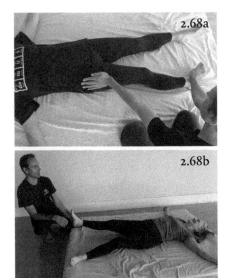

2.68a

2.68b

Chop-chop: Bring your palms together. Separate your fingers, keep them loose, and chop down all along the leg.

Transition: to **Lunge.**

Scoop the client's thigh with your hands and shake and jostle the leg up or down against the floor.

Scoot down to the client's foot. Grasp over their ankle and traction the leg.

Finish by brushing your hands down the leg.

Transition: Begin the sequence from the top, on the other side.

Supine—Abdomen

Abdominal Massage relaxes the muscles in and around the abdominal cavity, often releasing lower back tension. It promotes general relaxation, stimulates digestion, and removes tension and blood stagnation in the abdominal organs. It is common for the recipient to experience the need to use the bathroom during or after this work. Encourage your clients to speak up about this before and during the treatment.

Even though Abdominal Massage is presented here as the next sequence, it is best performed right before working on the psoas. After **Step 63** ("lower back reset"), you may choose to transition into Abdominal Massage as follows.

Step 69. Sun and Moon stroke

Abdominal area warm-up.

Hands are curved up to keep them flat for easier gliding.

The movement is performed in the clockwise direction to go with the direction of peristalsis.

The bottom hand makes a full circle (Sun)—my left hand in the photos.

The top hand makes a crescent or semi-circle (Moon) around the transverse colon (top right to top left).

Repeat 8–10 times.

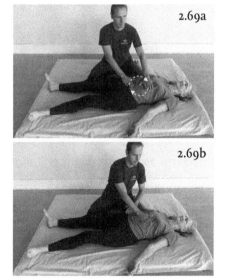

2.69a

2.69b

Step 70. Push-and-pull stroke

Hand over hand push and pull toward the navel.

Keep your hands flat for easier gliding.

Push with the heels of your palms.

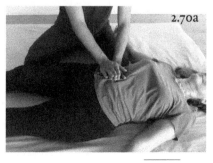

2.70a

Hook your fingers on the opposite side of the client's abdomen and pull to the center.

Repeat 8–10 times. Return to this technique in between other ones.

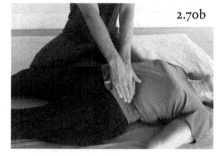

2.70b

Step 71. Releasing the "four corners"

Hold hand over hand.

Press directly against the bones into the muscle attachments.

Use fingerpads, not fingertips.

"Bone clean"—cross-fiber friction and circle in place: against the anterior iliac crests and against the lower ribs.

Move clockwise from your nearest side.

Application: Releases the attachments of the **obliques** and **transverse abdominis**.

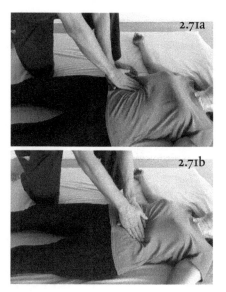

2.71a

2.71b

Step 72. Abdominal palm compressions

Perform six steady and deep palm compressions (see **Diagram 21**).

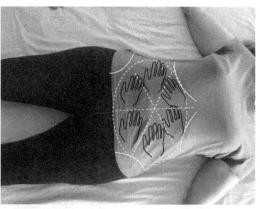

Diagram 21. Abdominal palm compressions

Move clockwise, starting at the bottom right (at the ascending colon).

Sink on the exhale, hold for one or two breaths, release on the inhale.

Go around once.

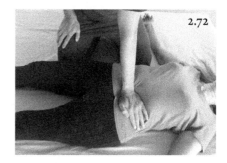

Step 73. Small intestine stimulation

Use the back of your hand and circle quickly and lightly over the navel.

This technique warms and stimulates blood flow.

Go at one circle per second or faster.

Perform 20–30 circles, or until you feel the area warming up.

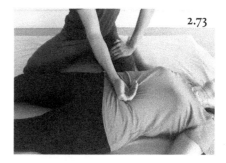

Step 74. Abdominal points

Transition: to **Lunge.**

Press with thumbs or thumb over thumb.

Press down on the exhale, hold for one or two breaths, and release on the inhale.

Follow the points in order (see **Diagram 22**).

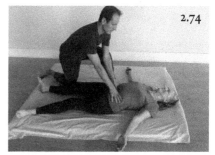

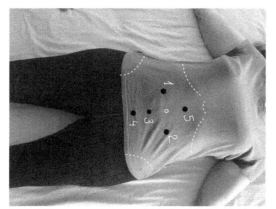

Diagram 22. Abdominal points for relaxation and digestive stimulation

It is normal to feel the abdominal artery pulse, especially on Points 3, 4, and 5.

Application: Stimulates digestion, releases abdominal organ tension.

Traditional Chinese Medicine reference:

- Points 1 and 2: Stomach 25 (ST25) (to improve digestion)

- Point 3: Conception Vessel 12 (CV12) (relaxation)

- Point 4: CV6 (vitality)

- Point 5: CV4 (vitality).

Refer to **Diagram 3** for other acupressure points.

"Make nice" with push and pull and Sun and Moon strokes.

Supine—Arms and Shoulders

Step 75. Arm traction

Transition C: Lunge to **One-Leg-Out.**

Lean on your arm and sit down.

Sit far enough to traction and extend the client's arm fully. Grasp at the wrist.

Avoid "skin burn" on the wrist.

Pull and release in a wave-like motion 5–6 times.

Do not yank!

Instead, extend the client's arm smoothly so they feel a gentle traction in all three joints: wrist, elbow, and shoulder.

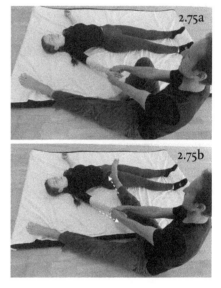

Variation: Foot press and traction. Place your lower heel (extended leg) into the **gluteus medius**.

Press your heel and pull the client's arm as above, 5–6 times.

Avoid "skin burn" at the wrist.

Step 76. Wrist decompression

A. Thumb press. Anchor and stretch the fascia across the wrist joint from the hand toward the forearm.

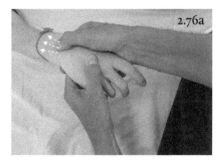

B. Press your thumbs over the wrist. Traction gently and mobilize the wrist.

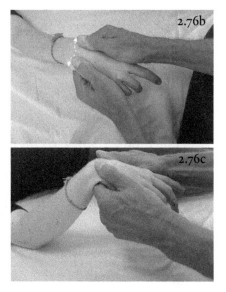

C. Thumb glide. Glide out and flex the wrist at the same time. Repeat 5–6 times.

Step 77. Opening hand channels

Before treating the arm and shoulder, it is important to open the hand energy channels so energy can flow and restrictions or blockages released in the arm or shoulder are not blocked at the wrist and hand.

Begin in the center of the wrist.

Thumb circle into the wrist tendons and carpal/metacarpal bones. Strum over them (see **Diagram 23**).

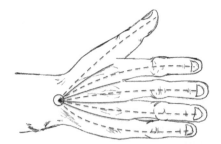

Diagram 23. Hand sen lines

Thumb circle over each line.

Note the 4 lines between the bones and the 5 lines over the bones.

On the lines between the bones, dig in to release tension.

On the bone lines, go out to each fingertip.

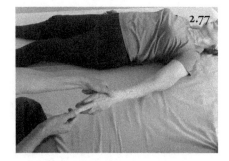

Squeeze at the fingertip between your thumb and index finger and quickly pull up to make a "pop" sound.

Step 78. Palmar lines and fascia

There are 5 lines on the palmar surface (see **Diagram 24**).

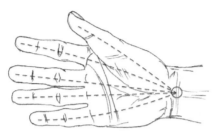

Diagram 24. Palm sen lines

Lift the client's forearm so that their palm is facing you.

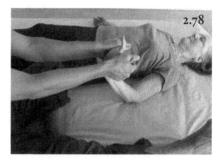

Support the back of their hand and fingers with your fingers. Press and slide your thumbs from the heel of the palm out to each fingertip.

Repeat 2–3 times.

Step 79. Wrist rotation and flexion

Interlace your fingers with the client's, hold at the wrist, flex their knuckles, pull and rotate their hand at the wrist.

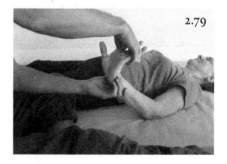

Flex their wrist forward and back and side to side.

Step 80. Opening forearm channels

Next, we must free up energy flow in the forearms.

There are two lines on the inside of the forearm (medial or ventral surface), and two lines on the outside (lateral or dorsal) (see **Diagrams 25a and 25b**).

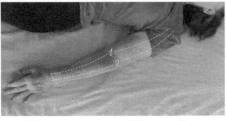

Diagram 25a. Lateral forearm lines

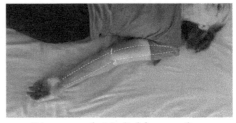

Diagram 25b. Medial forearm lines

Each line follows the two bones of the forearm: the ulna and the radius.

Outside line 1: Radius (thumb side) matches the Large Intestine Meridian in Traditional Chinese Medicine.

Outside line 2: Ulna (pinky-finger side).

Inside line 1: Radius.

Inside line 2: Ulna.

Outside lines 1 and 2: Hold at the client's wrist. Thumb circle and thumb strum over "ropey" muscles.

Start at the elbow and move down 2–3 times each line.

Press to the bones!

Muscles: Brachioradialis, forearm extensors.

Inside lines 1 and 2: Thumb circle and thumb strum.

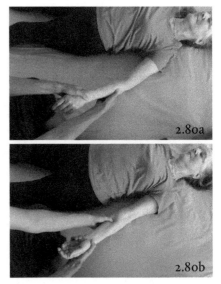

Start at the elbow and move down 2–3 times each line.

Press to the bones.

Muscles: Biceps brachii attachments, forearm flexors, pronator teres.

Transition: Tripod. Lean on your arm to lift up.

Step 81. Inside arm press

Bring the client's arm out, palm up.

A: Palm press from wrist to shoulder 2–3 times.

Use your body weight to press. Rock in and out. Press and hold compressions as needed.

B: Knee press. On the forearm only (not the upper arm)!

Keep your hands on the floor for support.

Knee press and release, rocking in to press, 1–2–3–2–1.

Stay away from the elbow.

Variation C: Foot press. Standing up, use the medial arch of your inside foot. Rock in and out.

Press and turn your foot in (invert) for deeper compressions.

Work from the wrist to the shoulder, skipping over the elbow.

Caution: Be careful *not* to press on the medial humerus under the biceps brachii, the site of the median and ulnar nerves.

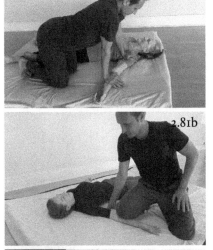

2.81a

2.81b

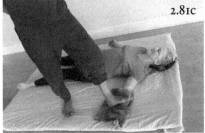

2.81c

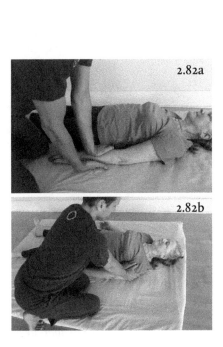

Step 82. Outside (lateral) arm press

Bring the client's arm alongside their body, palm down. Cup their forearm between your hands.

Rock in and out to press or squeeze their forearm.

Go up and down 2–3 times.

Skip the elbow.

Bring your fingers under the client's upper arm. Place your thumbs on top.

Rock in and out.

Press or squeeze the arm.

2.82a

2.82b

Caution: Do not press down on the client's upper arm without the support of your fingers underneath, or you may push their arm out of its socket!

Variation: Knee press. Forearm only (not upper arm)!

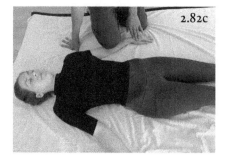

Apply pressure gradually. Rock in and out.

Move from the elbow to the wrist.

Address the **brachioradialis**.

CLINICAL FOCUS #7: CARPAL TUNNEL SYNDROME

The carpal tunnel is the pathway of nerves and tendons running on the medial side of the wrist. Some people have a narrower carpal tunnel than others. This narrower tunnel has the potential to restrict those nerves, inflaming the tendons, especially when combined with activities that create tension in the forearm flexor muscles (for example, keyboard typing and tennis). This restriction, or compression, of the nerves and subsequent aggravation and inflammation of tendons is known as carpal tunnel syndrome. It is accompanied by pain, weakness, and inflammation in the wrist.

It is the median nerve that gets compressed (see **Diagram 26**) under the flexor retinaculum, also known as the transverse carpal ligament. The sensation of pain and weakness may also be felt in the first three fingers (thumb, index, and middle) because the median nerve extends down them.

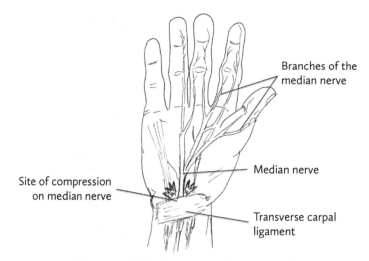

Diagram 26. Median nerve wrist compression

Additionally, the median nerve may get entrapped high on the forearm, under a tight pronator teres muscle (see **Diagram 27**).

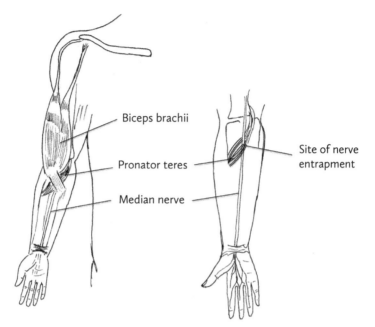

Diagram 27. Median nerve forearm entrapment

Carpal tunnel protocol

Perform wrist decompression, as in **Step 76**, and follow the steps through hand and palm lines. Thumb glide over the flexor retinaculum to loosen it up.

Thumb-strip and cross-fiber friction the **pronator teres** and **forearm flexors** in multiple strips (lines) (same technique as **Step 80**) and open the forearm channels. Cross-fiber friction at the origin, middle, and insertion of the **pronator**.

Transition: Tabletop/Tripod.

Knee press, or double-thumb press, over tight points—pronator, biceps' distal tendon and bicipital aponeurosis, and flexor muscles. Press and rock in place with your knee along the length of the forearm, as in **Step 81, "B."**

CLINICAL FOCUS #8: BRACHIAL PLEXUS NERVE ENTRAPMENT

The arm is enervated by the spinal nerves exiting out of cervical vertebrae C2–C7. This bundle of nerves runs between the clavicle and the ribs (thoracic outlet), and is generally called the brachial plexus of nerves.

There are several muscles that may entrap or compress this bundle of nerves, causing pain, numbness, and loss of function (weakness) in the arm. These are the scalenes, pectoralis minor, subclavius, and subscapularis (see **Diagram 28**). All four muscles and their related tissues should be treated to resolve a nerve entrapment.

The pectoralis minor is the most common culprit of the brachial plexus entrapment. It attaches on ribs 3, 4, and 5. When chronically tight, this powerful little muscle compresses the nerves that run underneath (**Diagram 28**). The scalenes (anterior, middle, and posterior) attach to ribs 1 and 2. When tight, these neck muscles may pull up on the ribs, narrowing the thoracic outlet and compressing the nerves. A tight subclavius may cause the same issue as it connects the clavicle to rib 1. The subscapularis is a thick rotator cuff muscle—it does not compress the spinal nerves directly. However, it attaches to the front of the scapula and the arm bone (humerus)—its fibers lie under the brachial plexus nerves. When tight or scarred from overuse (like pitching a ball or wrestling), these subscapularis fibers may push up on the nerves, or, in rare cases, entwine with the spinal nerves.

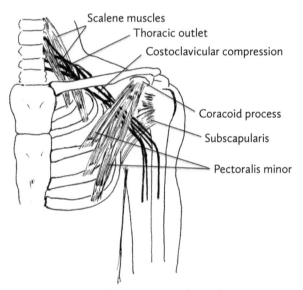

Diagram 28. Brachial plexus nerves and muscles

The following sequence is the protocol to treat these muscles and other related tissues to release the nerve entrapment.

1. Release the **pectoralis minor** with **Step 83** below. Cross-fiber friction at the coracoid process attachment. Grasp and squeeze the muscle looking for TPs. Cross-fiber friction the pectoralis minor attachments on ribs 3-5—"bone clean" ribs 3-5—press against the ribs to search for TPs. The most common pectoralis minor TPs are near the attachments on the ribs.

2. Cross-fiber friction the **subscapularis** attachment on the arm. Refer to **Clinical focus #9** on the **rotator cuff** for details. Abduct the arm to 45 degrees and rotate it externally as much as is comfortable for the client. Thumb press or finger press straight to the head of the humerus.

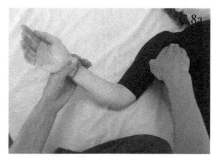

3. Cross-fiber and with-fiber friction against the bone. Repeat at different angles of the arm abduction and external rotation.

4. Perform **Steps 84–87** below, releasing the rest of the **subscapularis** and related tissues.

5. In side-lying position, pull the client's arm in front of their shoulder (Photo C.8b). This opens the space behind the clavicle and makes the **subclavius** more accessible. Lunge over the client's head with your upper foot. "Bone clean" over and under the clavicle (Photo C.8c). If open, grasp the clavicle between your thumb and index finger and "bone clean" the **subclavius** on the posterior aspect of the bone. It may be tender!

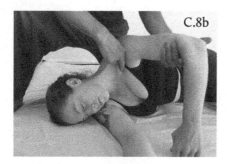

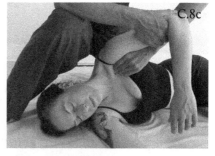

6. Grasp around the clavicle with the index fingers of both hands—one from the superior angle and the other from the inferior angle. Cross-fiber friction and pinch-and-roll the **subclavius**.

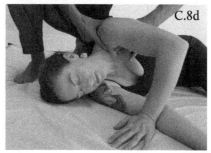

7. In side-lying position, perform **Step 151**, thumb gliding over the **scalenes** (Photos C.8e and C.8f). Cross-fiber friction and hold for TPs.

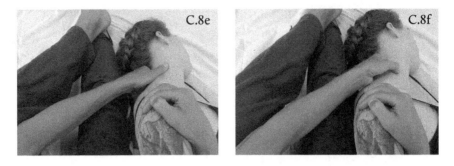

8. Perform **Step 157** ("pectoralis treatment" in side-lying position).

9. It may also be helpful to work on the **scalenes** one more time in the supine position.

10. Refer to **Clinical focus #17** on the **scalenes** for details.

Step 83. Pectoralis release

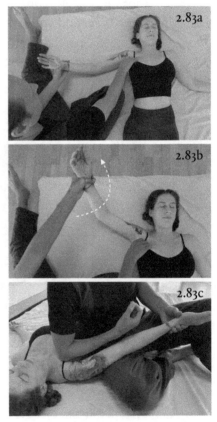

Transition: Hold the client's wrist with your outside hand, lean on your inside hand, and scoot in to reach their pectoral muscles.

Finger press the client's pectoralis area with your fingerpads to warm it up.

Grasp and roll the pectoralis fibers between your thumb and fingers.

Cross-fiber friction against the sternum.

"Pin and stretch"—grasp over the pectoralis muscle bundle with your thumb and fingers.

Squeeze and stretch the client's arm out using your outside hand (hold their wrist).

Compress the **pectoralis minor** attachments against ribs 3, 4, and 5. Hold these compressions for 5–6 seconds.

Variation: Elbow press. Scoot in under the client's arm, holding their wrist. Place your elbow under the coracoid process.

Allow the weight of your elbow to melt into the pectoralis attachments (Wind Gate point).

Hold for 5–6 seconds; reposition a few times.

Hold the wrist and gently move the client's arm up or down and side to side during compressions.

Step 84. Underarm release

Transition: Scoot up in **One-Leg-Out** to bring your straight leg above the client's head (Photo 2.84a) or lift up to **Tripod**.

Techniques:

A. Bring the client's arm alongside their ear and stretch their arm up gently.

B. Palm press down the side (along the ribcage and lateral border of the scapula).

C. Finger press and circle and thumb press and circle along the lateral border of the scapula, **triceps**, **latissimus**, **teres**, and **subscapularis** (also see **Clinical focus #9** on **rotator cuff** treatment).

Muscles: Latissimus, serratus anterior, infraspinatus, teres major and minor, sub-scapularis, triceps.

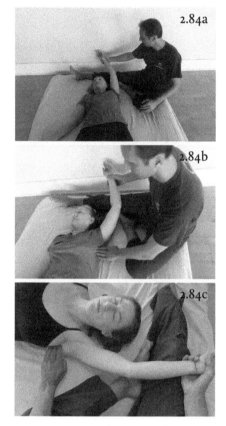

Step 85. Scapula cradle

Positioning is important for the efficacy of these techniques: Slide your *upper hand* under the client's scapula and hook your fingers on the medial border.

Bend your upper knee and rest the client's arm over your upper leg (between your knee and shoulder).

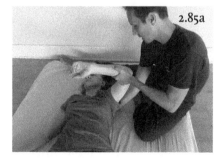

Techniques: Your upper hand stays under the scapula. Pop your fingers up into the muscles between the scapula and the spine.

Use your lower hand to:

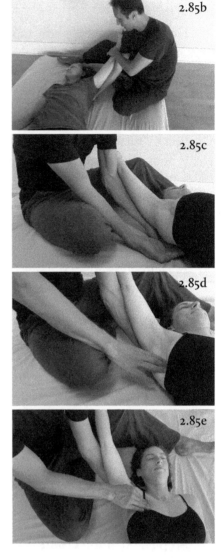

2.85b

2.85c

2.85d

- Help the upper hand to traction the scapula.

- Finger walk along the spine and the medial border.

- Finger circle along the lateral edge of the scapula.

- Finger press into the **subscapularis**.

See also **Clinical focus #9** on the **rotator cuff**.

Muscles: Rhomboids, mid trapezius, levator scapula, erector spinae, infraspinatus, subscapularis.

Variation: "Pain sandwich." Keep your upper hand underneath, cupping the client's scapula.

2.85e

With your lower hand, finger press on the pectoralis muscles and rib attachments in the front.

Cup your hands over and under and gently jostle the shoulder.

Step 86. Shoulder grasping

Bring the client's arm down. Grasp over their **upper trapezius** and **supraspinatus** with your upper hand.

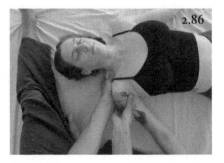

2.86

Grasp over their **deltoids** with your lower hand. Use the middle finger of your upper hand to "bone clean" the **supraspinatus**.

Pluck "the strings" of the **anterior deltoid** with the thumb of your lower hand.

CLINICAL FOCUS #9: ROTATOR CUFF MUSCLES

The shoulder joint affords a wonderful range of motion at the expense of its own stability. The glenoid fossa is the concave surface of the joint, rimmed with a ring-like fibrocartilage (the glenoid labrum), providing an articular surface, but not much support.

The task of support in the glenohumeral joint falls to the soft tissue structure called the rotator cuff—the four SITS muscles (from front to back, the acronym should really be SSIT: **subscapularis, supraspinatus, infraspinatus,** and **teres minor**) and their combined tendon attachments around the head of the humerus (see **Diagram 29**).

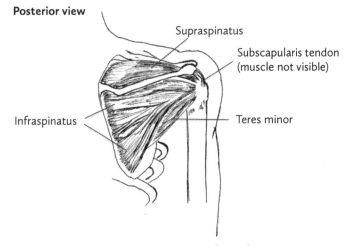

Diagram 29. Rotator cuff muscles

The main task of these muscles is to anchor the head of the humerus into the glenoid fossa, and they must do it constantly. In any standing or sitting position where the arm is not supported by external means (like an armrest), the joint depends on the activity of these muscles. Secondly, whenever there is movement at the shoulder, these four muscles orchestrate a complex gliding and rotating motion that stabilizes the joint throughout its range.

Problems arise due to weakness and when these tendons are placed under a heavy, or constant, load. An area just proximal to the greater tubercle attachment is termed the "critical zone" (see **Diagram 30**) where long periods of ischemia lead to atrophy and degeneration of the tendon fibers. This is the most likely spot for tendon tears to occur.

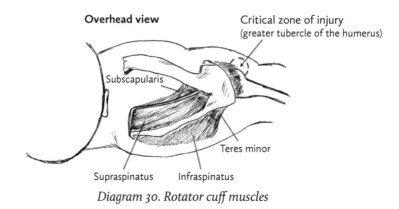

Diagram 30. Rotator cuff muscles

Furthermore, other tendons, bursas, and the joint capsule fill this small space between the head of the humerus and the overhanging acromion process. They are easily injured by poor biomechanics, overuse, and repetitive motion. Left unattended, the lesions around the rotator cuff will compound and may eventually lead to "frozen shoulder."

Subscapularis

The subscapularis is a powerful muscle. Its tendon can be palpated between the bicipital groove and the coracoid process (see **Diagram 31**). It is the primary medial rotator of the humerus, and is involved in actions like throwing a ball, swimming, tennis serves, and opening the lid of a jar (right-handed).

A total of 75–80 percent of all throwing injuries involve the subscapularis. Pitchers are particularly susceptible. Minor tears don't draw much attention because the muscle is so strong. But one after another tears build up with scar tissue, shortening and weakening the muscle. A sudden exertion causes a more serious tear and considerable pain and disability.

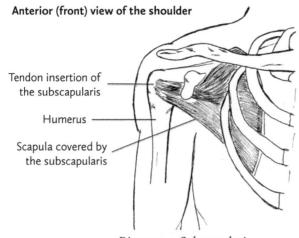

Diagram 31 Subscapularis

A sure indication of a subscapularis injury is that resisted medial rotation causes pain. Have your client resist against your hand on their medial shoulder rotation (their elbow tucked in by the side). Other medial rotators (latissimus, pectoralis major, and teres major) are mainly adductors, so when resisted adduction causes no pain, these muscles can be ruled out.

There are two places where the subscapularis can be accessible: the tendon insertion at the humerus and the lateral fibers on the anterior surface of the scapula (accessible by drawing out the scapula). Both of these techniques have been covered in the previous few steps. Here they are again, for easy reference.

TENDON INSERTION

In supine position, abduct the arm to 30–45 degrees and rotate it externally as much as is comfortable for the client.

Thumb press or finger press straight to the head of the arm bone—the insertion site of the subscapularis on the lesser tubercle, just medial to the bicipital groove.

Cross-fiber and with-fiber friction against the bone—up or down and side to side, for 30 seconds.

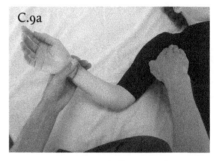
C.9a

Repeat at different angles of the arm abduction and external rotation.

Loosen the arm and shoulder between rounds with gentle jostling and grasping.

ANTERIOR SURFACE OF THE SCAPULA

This technique is the same as **Step 85** (finger press into the subscapularis).

Working on the client's left side, cradle the scapula with your right hand underneath (the "pain sandwich" move) and traction it out. This traction makes the lateral fibers of the subscapularis more accessible.

Use your left hand to press into the subscapularis. Cross-fiber friction over accessible fibers.

Examine for TPs. Use the fingers or thumb.

Caution: Do not press high in the axilla to avoid hitting the axillary nerve bundle.

Supraspinatus

The supraspinatus originates on the supraspinous fossa of the scapula and inserts on the superior facet of the greater tubercle of the humerus (see **Diagram 29**). Because of this location, it plays a key role in holding the head of the humerus in the glenoid fossa. It also initiates abduction of the humerus before deltoids take over.

The supraspinatus is one of the most active and most commonly injured rotator cuff muscles from acute or chronic overuse and repetitive motion. About 70 percent of rotator cuff injuries are in the supraspinatus. It has a relatively thin tendon, compared to the other four muscles, that runs under the acromion. This tendon gets pinched, and rubbed raw, between the acromion and the humerus. If frayed or scarred, it gets thickened with scar tissue and swollen with inflammation, causing the infamous "frozen shoulder" condition.

The supraspinatus is stressed by holding the arms up (hairstylists), or holding the arms overhead (painters, plumbers). Tennis players use the supraspinatus with every serve. It can be injured by bracing yourself from a fall. It is strained by carrying luggage at your side and trying to keep the bags from banging against your leg.

Indication: Resisted abduction causes pain. Have your client lift their arm out to the side against your resistance.

Treatment must address the attachment on the humerus, the tendon near the acromion, and the belly of the muscle lying in the supraspinous fossa. The supraspinatus can be worked on in any position: supine, prone, side, and seated. Here are some common techniques.

Supine: Grasp over the upper trapezius.

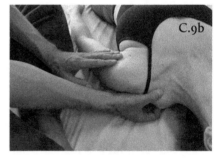

C.9b

Place your thumb on the attachment at the humerus (superior aspect of the greater tubercle).

Place your index and middle fingers on the muscle above the spine of the scapula.

Thumb press the attachment.
Finger press the muscle against the bone.
Compress to examine for TPs.
Cross-fiber and with-fiber friction.
Start at the superior angle of the scapula and move out toward the acromion.
Use your index finger to pulse or flush into the "dusty corner," the corner of the acromion.

Prone: In **Lunge**, grasp over the trapezius and thumb press into the supraspinatus, compressing it against the bone. Brace your elbow against your knee for more pressure.

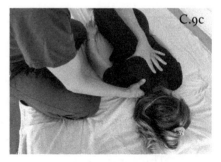

C.9c

Cross-fiber friction and examine for TPs. Look for stringy, taut bands.

Treat the "dusty corner" and the tendon within it—flush it with compressions.

Infraspinatus and teres minor

Both of these muscles perform the same action (external shoulder rotation) and are susceptible to similar patterns of tension and injury. They both insert on the posterior aspect of the greater tubercle of the humerus (see **Diagram 29**). Abduct the arm to 90 degrees and support it to feel the tendon of the infraspinatus just below the lateral edge of the acromion. The teres minor lies slightly inferior.

They are both involved in actions like putting on a shirt, reaching behind into the back of a car, writing, and backhand movements in racket sports. They are not particularly strong muscles, and are easily overwhelmed by stronger internal rotators (subscapularis, pectoralis major), and get ischemic and develop TPs.

Indication: Resisted external rotation causes pain. Elbow tucked in by their side, have the client push against your resistance as they rotate their arm back. If pain is also felt on the abduction with external rotation, the lesion lies at the distal end of the infraspinatus tendon, on the greater tubercle.

As with other muscles, there are many techniques of treating the infraspinatus and teres minor.

Supine: Perform flat muscle compressions on the infraspinatus, as in **Step 85** above ("scapula cradle"), and specifically the "pain sandwich" technique. Press your fingers up and cross-fiber friction on the scapula (look for nodules and depressions) and cross-fiber friction on the tendon under the lateral aspect of the spine of the scapula.

Prone: Bring the client's arm up (Photo C.9d), or out to at least 45 degrees, so that the lateral border of the scapula becomes easily accessible.

Compress around the scapula.

Cross-fiber friction on the **infraspinatus**—examine for TPs on the scapula, look for nodules that feel like "speed bumps."

For the **teres minor**, compress against the lateral border of the scapula and hold for TPs.

Infraspinatus tendon: Friction on the tendon near its attachment on the humerus (Photo C.9e). Find the tendon just below (inferior to) the angle where the spine of the scapula turns into the acromion process. The tendon is wide and thick and about an inch long from the musculotendinous junction to the insertion. Cross-fiber and with-fiber friction. At the distal end, deep friction parallel to the shaft of the humerus (Photo C.9f).

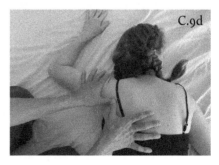
C.9d

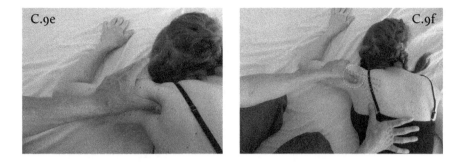

Step 87. Triceps release

Transition: to **Hero.** Bring your knees together and sit on your heels with your inside knee right next to the client's shoulder, facing toward the client's feet.

Pick up the client's arm at the wrist, raise it, and rest it alongside your thigh.

Techniques: Thumb walk the length of the triceps 2–3 times.

Treat distal and proximal attachments by strumming across (cross-fiber friction) at the olecranon process and infraglenoid tubercle.

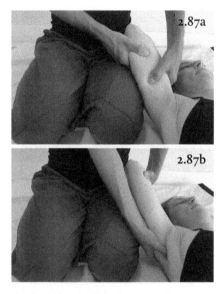

Step 88. The "waiter's tray" stretch

Transition: to **Tripod.** Move over to the client's side.

Bring the client's arm into the *"waiter's tray"* position—bend the client's fingers back so that they point toward their shoulder and plant their hand 2–3 inches away from their head.

Press gently over their triceps and the iliac crest.

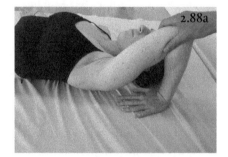

Grasp and squeeze over the triceps.

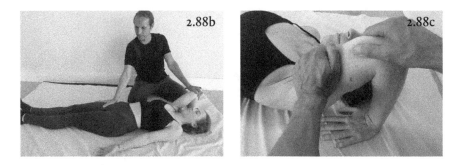

Step 89. Overhead traction

Hold the client by the wrist and move over the client's head.

Traction and shake their arm alongside the ear 4–5 times.

Rest their arm alongside the body or on the abdomen.

After finishing both sides, grasp both wrists and traction the client's arms at the same time.

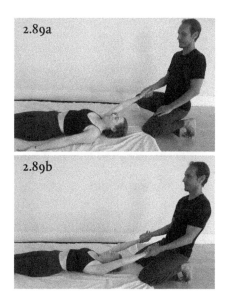

Prone—Lower Body

Step 90. Foot walk on medial arches

First, press with the balls of your feet.

Start with light pressure, facing the client.

Rock foot to foot. Modify pressure as needed.

Focus on the medial arches, not the toes or heels.

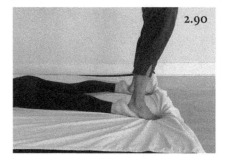

2.90

Variation: Facing backward. Use your heels. Keep most of your weight on the balls of your feet and apply more pressure only if the client is comfortable.

Step 91. Achilles tendon squeeze

Transition: to **Hero** or **Tripod.**

Grasp the Achilles tendon between the thumb and fingers and pull up along the length of the tendon.

Repeat 2–3 times.

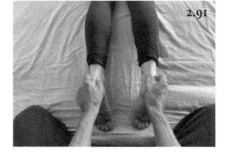

2.91

Step 92. Double ankle dorsiflexion

While squeezing the tendon at the heel, lift the client's lower legs, place your forearms over their feet, and press down into dorsiflexion.

Drop your elbow as low as you can.

Press and hold for 2 seconds 3 times, each time deeper.

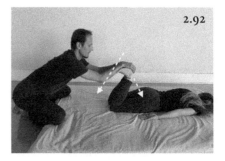

2.92

Step 93. Double knee flexion

Switch your hand position to hold under the client's feet.

Transition: to **Lunge.**

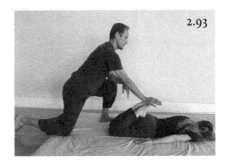

Cross the client's feet at the toe mounts (not the ankles!).

Press over their toes—heels to tailbone.

Press and hold for 3–4 seconds 3 times, each time deeper.

Re-cross the feet and repeat.

Step 94. Plantar fascia treatment

Plantar fasciitis may also be treated from this position (see **Clinical focus #1**). Or simply follow these techniques to "warm up" the fascia.

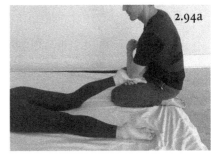

Transition: sit back to **Hero** or **Tripod.**

A. Elbow press. Rest the client's right foot over your inside knee (left).

Slide your right hand under their foot to support it.

Press and roll your inside elbow and forearm into the foot.

Elbow circle on foot points.

B. "Pin and stretch"—hold the client's foot with your thumbs on top and fingers underneath.

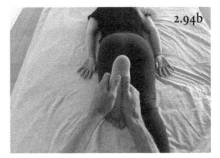

Anchor your thumbs into the fascia under the heel and flex the ankle.

Repeat 8–10 times, repositioning at different spots along the bands of tissue.

Flex and circle the ankle in both directions. Pull, shake, and let go of the foot.

Switch sides.

CLINICAL FOCUS #10 (OPTIONAL): ACHILLES TENDINITIS

You may choose to treat Achilles tendinitis in this position.

Use cross-fiber friction along the fibers and look for the sensitive nodule of the tendon tear (the bulge in the tissue).

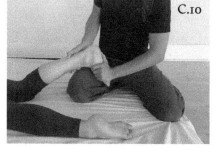

C.10

Often, it is even more effective to provide treatment from both positions: a short treatment (5–10 minutes) in supine, as shown earlier, and another short treatment in prone. This in-between break gives the injured tissues "time to breathe" and to assimilate the benefits of the focused work.

Switch sides.

Step 95. Palm walk lower legs

Transition: to **Tabletop.**

Palm walk, rocking side to side.

Up–down–up–down.

Keep your back in Lazy-Cat Back.

Lean with your body weight.

Keep your fingers turned out.

Keep your arms straight at 90 degrees.

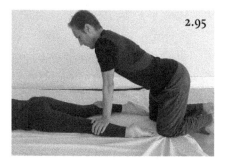

2.95

Step 96. Lower leg inside lines

Transition: to **Hero.**

Sit between the client's feet.

Thumb walk side to side, up and down.

Move 1 inch at a time.

Line 1: Press along the tibia. Start right next to the medial malleolus.

Press in and pull away from the bone.

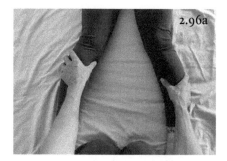

2.96a

Line 2: Start on the medial aspect of the Achilles tendon.

Press into the tissue along the medial head of the gastrocnemius.

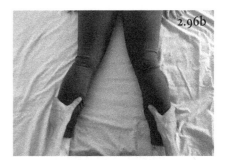

Step 97. Knee points circle

Thumb circle over the knee crease 8–10 times with light pressure.

3 points: Medial, center, lateral.

If sensing a pulse, do not press deeply.

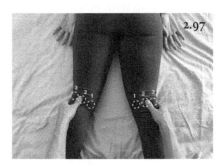

Step 98. Palm walk upper legs

Transition: step up to **Lunge.**

Palm walk, rocking side to side, up to the ischial tuberosities. Up–down 3–4 times.

Lean with your body weight.

Keep your fingers turned out.

Keep your arms straight at 90 degrees.

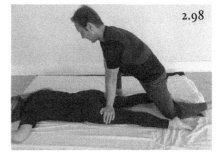

Step 99. Medial upper legs lines

Thumb walk side to side, up and down.

Move 1 inch at a time.

Line 1: Medial—continuous with line 1 on the lower leg—medial knee (adductor attachments) up along the adductor longus to the pubic bone.

Go up only as far as comfortable—stop 1.5–2 inches before the pubic attachments.

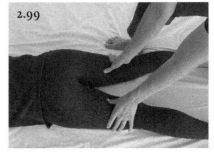

Line 2: Continuous with line 2 on the lower leg, running between the hamstrings and adductors.

Step 100. Hamstrings knee press

Caution: This technique is only appropriate for clients who are comfortable to handle over 50 percent of your weight.

Transition: Tabletop.

Stand up with your feet together between the client's knees, or with your feet on the outside of the client's knees.

Bring your hands to the floor and lower your knees onto the client's hamstrings under the ischial tuberosities.

Technique: Keep half your weight on your arms.

Anchor your feet with toes under.

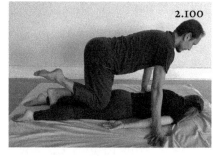

2.100

Work one side at a time—move your knee side to side to cross-fiber friction the hamstrings.

Move up and down to address different spots.

Switch knees as needed.

Step 101. Ischial tuberosity knee press with back palm press

Step up and place your knees right under the ischial tuberosities.

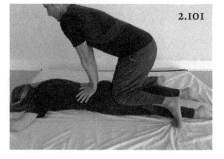

2.101

Place your hands, fingers pointing out, at the sides of the client's sacrum.

Rock in to apply pressure; rock out to release.

Keep your arms straight at right angles, with Lazy-Cat Back.

Palm press up the back to the thoracic area and back.

Step 102. Gluteal knee compressions

This is a 5–6-second straight-down kneeling compression.

Rock side to side slowly, if comfortable for the client. Keep your toes under for balance.

A. Under the ischial tuberosities.

B. In the middle of the gluteus maximus.

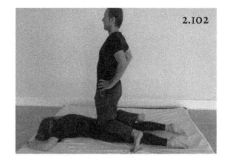

2.102

Prone—Back and Shoulders

Step 103. Gluteal knee press and back palm press

Place your knees in the center of the gluteus maximus, as in **Step 102, "B."**

Palm press from the sacrum to the upper corners of the scapulae.

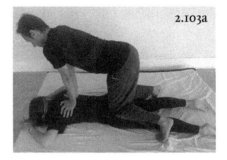
2.103a

Up and down 2 times.

Move 1 to 2 inches at a time.

Keep the rhythm slow—no faster than 2 seconds per compression.

Keep your palm pressure gentle at first; deepen if the client feels comfortable.

A. Knee roll. Roll your knees forward and back over the gluteals by lifting your feet.

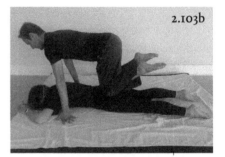
2.103b

B. Calf slap. Quickly bounce your feet on the client's calves.

Make sure to get a good balance first—your hands on the floor or on the client's back.

Step 104. Back press

Position: Kneeling on the glutes, or **Lunge** over the client.

After palm pressing the back in **Step 103**, we can use thumbs to go over the Sen lines.

A. Thumb press or thumb circle up and down the back, moving one vertebra at a time.

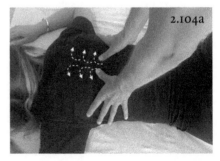
2.104a

Line 1: Thumbs right next to the spine (right off the spinous processes) (see **Diagram 32**).

Line 2: Thumbs in the lamina groove (about 1 inch off the spine).

B. Knuckle press, or knuckle roll upward— from the sacrum—and go to T1 vertebra, 2–3 times.

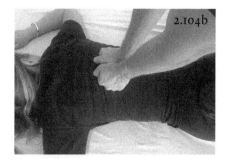

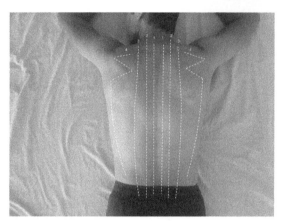

Diagram 32. Back sen lines

Step 105. Back warming with palm circles

Transition: to **Tripod.**

Step down to either side.

Palm circle both sides of the back with broad circles.

2–3 rounds up and down.

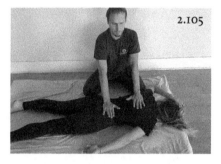

Step 106. Back lines 1–2–3 diagnostic

Technique: "Thumb chasing thumb" (press, pull, and catch up).

Start either at the top (C5–C6) or the sacral vertebrae (**Diagram 32**).

Go over each line once or twice.

Keep pressure light and move 1 inch at a time, vertebra to vertebra.

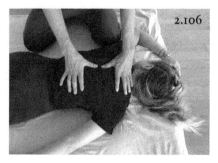

Start with **line 1:** Feel for any irregularities along the spine—dips, protrusions of vertebrae, crunchy ligaments, ropey muscles.

Line 2: Press into the lamina groove.

Line 3 runs deep along the transverse processes and off the medial border of the scapula, right off the edge of the quadratus lumborum and over the sacroiliac ligaments. Tension and pain in the lower back can be addressed further with **Clinical focus #11** on **lower back pain**.

Step 107. Back elbow compressions

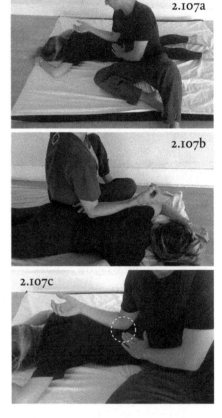

2.107a

2.107b

2.107c

Transition: sit in **Spiral**, **Sit-and-Lean**, or **Hero**.

Hero offers more height or leverage and is best for bigger clients.

Sit-and-Lean and **Spiral** positions may be more comfortable and best for working on the back for a longer period of time.

Note: Make sure to sit right next to the client's iliac spine and turn away from the client about 45 degrees.

Best tool: The "flat of the elbow"—2 inches of the ulna distal to the olecranon process (vs. the sharp "point of the elbow").

Use your outside hand to locate the spine.

Place your inside elbow off the spine at the iliolumbar ligament (**Diagram 33**).

Press and hold for 2–3 seconds.

Repeat compressions 4–5 times.

Move up along the spine 1 inch at a time.

Sink in *very* slowly. Move your forearm or elbow in place (with tissue) up and down a few times.

Note: Best to align your forearm parallel to the client's spine to avoid hitting the spinous processes.

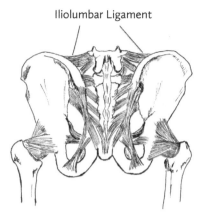

Iliolumbar Ligament

Diagram 33. Iliolumbar and sacral ligaments

Upon reaching the mid-back (T5–T6, aka "the bra line"), return to L1 and repeat 2–3 times.

Note: The client's arm may be in the "up" position, as in Photo 2.107a. If more comfortable, bring their arm to the down-sloping position, as in Photo 2.107d.

Variation: Mid- and upper back elbow compressions.

Transition: Tripod or Tabletop.

Upon reaching the mid-back, change your position to **Tripod** or **Tabletop**.

Perform the same-type compressions (sink and rock in place, up–down).

After one round of compressions along the mid-back, switch your elbows or forearms— use your upper arm and angle it along the client's spine, as in Photo 2.107e.

Perform several rounds of elbow or forearm compressions up to T1–C7, sliding off the shoulder over the upper trapezius.

To understand more about the pain patterns behind mid-back tension, see **Article 5** in the Appendix.

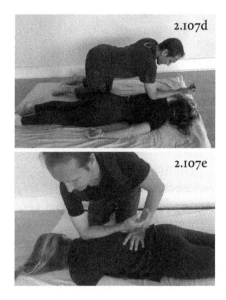

2.107d

2.107e

Step 108. Back double-elbow press

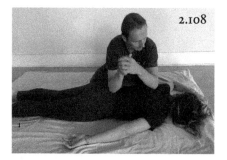

2.108

Transition: sit in **Low Tripod.**

Sink your elbows slowly and circle them in place.

Reposition and repeat.

Keep your back in Lazy-Cat Back position.

Caution: Do not press directly on the ribs or spine.

Variation: Roll glutes and latissimus. Place your *forearms* over the gluteus maximus and lattisimus attachments at the scapula.

Circle both sides at the same time.

Circle side to side and traction away from side to side.

CLINICAL FOCUS #11: LOWER BACK PAIN (FROM A DEEP MUSCLE PULL OR TEAR)

You're taking a shower and drop your soap. You reach down to pick it up, and pop! Something snaps in the lower back followed by sharp pain. Or you're sitting at your desk, and you drop your pen. You reach down and... There are a million ways a muscle pull can occur. It may occur while performing the most mundane task. Usually, it happens when the muscles are not warmed up and are already strained due to poor postural habits and overstretching. Healthy strong muscles are less likely to get pulled.

One of the most common injuries in the lower back is a pulled or torn **multifidus** or **rotatores** muscle (see **Diagram 34**). These muscles are short—connecting vertebra to vertebra—which is the reason for their high tendency for injuries—they don't have as much give as the longer superficial muscles. These are also the deepest muscles of the back. This is why the pain feels "really deep" and seems to radiate around the spine, often being mistaken for a bulging disc.

After the injury, the body constricts the tissues around a torn multifidus or rotatores to prevent further tissue tears, causing a localized spasm and stiffness, possibly leading to the infamous Pain–Spasm Cycle.

Over time, after four to eight weeks, the tear heals. The body lays a patch of collagen fibers (scar tissue) and the pain goes away. However, the scar tissue fibers are less elastic. The area is now less flexible and re-injury is more likely.

Clearly, it would be beneficial to break up those adhesions and reduce some of the internal scarring to maintain the health and mobility of these injured muscles. Cross-fiber friction techniques do exactly that—loosen the adhesions, remove the scar tissue, and restore healthy muscle function.

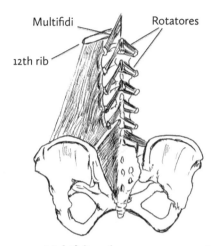

Diagram 34. Multifidi and rotatores – posterior view

After 24 hours past the injury, light cross-fiber friction can be applied to the injured muscles and surrounding tissues. Improved blood flow from the massage will help speed up recovery and healing.

After four to five days past the injury, the collagen bonds have been thickened, and deeper cross-fiber friction can be applied targeting those deep layers of multifidi and rotatores at the level of the transverse processes.

Thumb press to flush out, or elbow press, the iliolumbar ligament (see **Diagram 33** above). Often, this ligament is tender and full of scarred tissue, and is involved in supporting the lumbar spine and these muscles.

Continue to thumb-strip up–down into the deeper muscle layers (multifidi and rotatores).

Thumb press from the side (line 3), aiming for the transverse processes (Photo C.11).

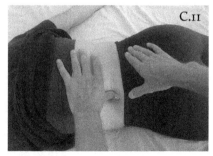

Always start with lighter strokes and deepen pressure if it is tolerated. Check in with the client.

Optional switch: Step over the client and repeat **Steps 106–108** on the other side.

CLINICAL FOCUS #12: SCIATICA

Sciatica is characterized by sharp pain shooting down the back of the leg. It is caused by a compressed nerve in a lumbar vertebra, usually L4 or L5. An intervertebral disc slips out (due to postural distortion, biomechanical overload, and/or ligament laxity) and presses on the spinal nerve (see **Diagram 35**). Sciatica can be intermittent or severe depending on the degree of the disc protrusion or bulging.

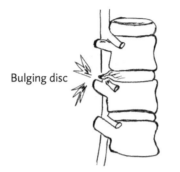

Bulging disc

Diagram 35. Bulging intervertebral disc

In severe cases, it may be treated via surgery. In most cases, however, the disc can be "convinced" to go back into its place. This may happen on its own by resting and relaxing the tissues surrounding the lumbar spine with Epsom salt baths, massage, and other relaxation methods.

I find that many sciatica sufferers prolong their recovery and exacerbate painful episodes by stretching the pain. This is a **strong contraindication**. If you suffer from sciatica, *whatever you do, do not stretch your lower back*. It will make it worse! Here is why:

The disc bulged out because of stretching, or another form of overloading.

Lower back muscles are chronically overstretched.

This may seem counter-intuitive because the lower back often "feels" tight. However, it feels tight precisely because it is overstretched.

What makes our lower back overstretched?

Sitting.

In today's world, we all sit too much. When we sit down, we stretch our lower backs. Muscles do not like to be stretched for too long. After a few minutes of sitting, the muscles of the back will begin to resist the continuous load of stretching. They will begin to contract themselves in self-protection. This innate response is known as **neural inhibition**—a protective mechanism of our body to avoid hurting itself. This is exactly why the back muscles "feel" tight.

Recommendations: To help these muscles, and ultimately prevent sciatica, avoid overstretching the lower back. Keep your posture upright, your lumbar spine in neutral or slightly arched (not rounded), when sitting for long periods of time.

Above all, keep your lower back muscles strong. This muscle strength keeps the intervertebral discs where they belong, between the vertebrae. If any discs bulge out, even if they do not cause any pain, strengthening the back muscles will push the discs back in. This is the real solution to sciatica: strength, not stretching.

Working on sciatica

- Release the **hamstrings**, **psoas**, and **piriformis**, as these muscles can cause sciatica-like back pain and symptoms.

- Perform with-fiber elbow compressions along the **erector spinae**, relaxing the muscles on both sides of the lumbar spine.

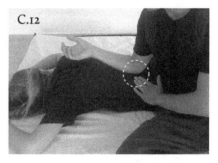

C.12

- Educate your clients about the importance of strengthening the lower back, and not stretching it (unless they do not sit and work out all the time).

Step 109. Shoulder press and squeeze

Transition: step up to **Lunge** (upper leg).

Bring the client's arm alongside their body.

Grasp over the client's shoulder with your upper hand.

Brace your elbow with your knee to *add more pressure and use less effort*, as in Photo 2.109.

Rock your body to use your body weight.

Squeeze and roll the muscles between your thumb and fingers, 8–10 times.

Muscles: Upper trapezius, supraspinatus, levator scapula.

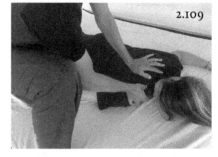

2.109

Step 110. Shoulder push–pull and circle

Techniques:

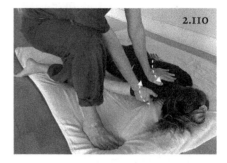

A. Push your lower hand into the client's **rhomboids**, while pulling up on the front of the shoulder 5–6 times.

B. Lift and circle the shoulder forward and back 3–4 times each direction.

Step 111. Pectoralis press in shoulder cradle, aka the "pain sandwich"

Transition: Hero or **Tripod**.

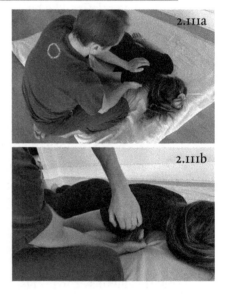

Sit next to the client's shoulder. Slide your upper hand under the client's shoulder to the **pectoralis** muscles or even to their sternum, if comfortable.

Point your fingerpads up toward the client's ribs 3–5 (**pectoralis minor** attachments).

Press your fingers into the pectoralis while simultaneously lifting the shoulder and pressing into the scapula or the **rhomboids** with your lower hand or thumb.

If hitting a sensitive trigger point on the pectoralis, hold it for 8–10 seconds.

Reposition your fingers and repeat 4–5 times.

Step 112. Scapula isolation in shoulder cradle

Keep your upper hand under the shoulder joint, as in **Step 111**.

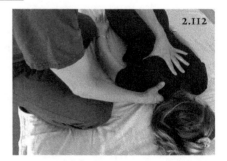

Grasp and lift the scapula with your other hand.

Check if the scapula is mobile and able to lift off the back.

Step 113. Scapula pull and rhomboid treatment

Position: stay in **Tripod**; or **Optional Transition:** to **Lunge** (Photo 2.113b).

Prop up the client's shoulder with your outside hand and hook your fingers on the medial border of the scapula.

Pull up on the scapula along the medial border.

Use your thumb, fingers, knuckles, or *elbow* to press and pull the **rhomboids** off the medial border of the scapula.

Address the common **pain points** (X's) of the intersection of the **lower trapezius** and **rhomboids**. Press and hold the TPs. Cross-fiber friction to break up adhesions.

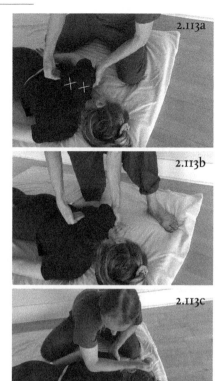

2.113a

2.113b

2.113c

Step 114. Arm press

Position: Tripod or **Hero**.

Scoot back a few inches to have room.

Palm press down the arm: **posterior deltoids**, **triceps**, forearm, wrist, and palm.

Repeat top–down 2–3 times.

Thumb press and thumb glide into the palm, focusing on the wrist, finger mounts, and the webbing of the thumb.

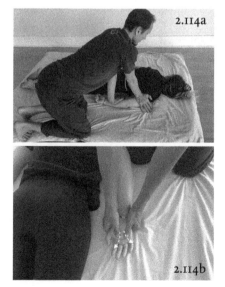

2.114a

2.114b

Step 115. Arm extension

Position: Tripod or **Hero.** Turn to face the client's side.

First, flex the wrist. Then lift the client's arm.

Be careful not to lift too fast or too far. Feel for the natural resistance in the arm joint.

Do not push past resistance. Hold for 2–3 seconds and repeat 2–3 times.

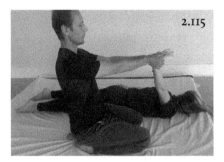

2.115

Step 116. "Arm lock" scapula release

From the arm extension in **Step 115**, fold the client's elbow behind their lower back into the "arm lock" position.

Scoot under the client's elbow with your lower knee.

Hold your upper hand underneath their shoulder.

Use your inside hand to do the same techniques as in **Step 113**, "scapula pull" (Photo 2.113a) and "rhomboid treatment" (Photos 2.113b and c).

Variation: Superior and inferior angles.

Tools: Thumb press and finger press.

Hold the TPs. Cross-fiber friction and "bone clean" over the spine of the scapula.

Muscles: Supraspinatus, levator scapula, trapezius, latissimus, serratus anterior.

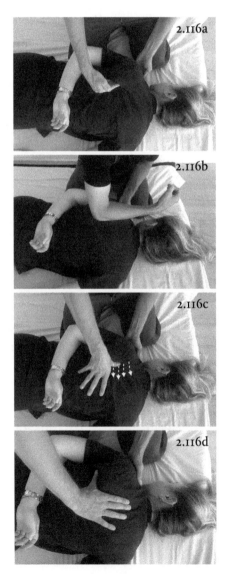

2.116a

2.116b

2.116c

2.116d

Step 117. Scapula lateral edge treatment

Positioning: Bring the client's arm around the floor into the "up" position to make the lateral border more available.

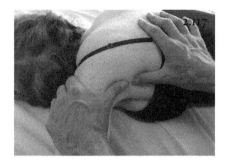

Thumb walk on the lateral border of the scapula.

Muscles: Teres major and minor, infraspinatus, serratus anterior, latissimus, triceps attachments at the infraglenoid tubercle.

If sensitive points are felt, slow down and hold thumb compressions.

Step 118. Latissimus and glutes foot press

Transition: Sit back and place your feet on the client's scapula attachment of the **latissimus dorsi** and on the **gluteus medius**.

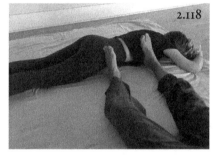

Walk your feet side to side, gently rocking the client's body and pushing compressions away from each other.

Step 119. Upper back overtop compressions

Transition: Tripod or **Sit-and-Lean.**

Slide up over the top of the client's shoulder.

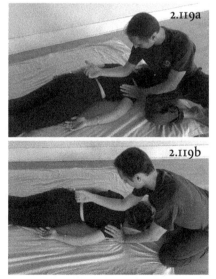

Muscles: Levator scapula, including its "crunchy" attachment at the superior angle of the scapula, upper trapezius, splenius capitis and cervicis.

In **Sit-and-Lean**, sit above the client's shoulder and use elbow press.

In **Tripod**, use elbow press, thumb press, and double-thumb press.

Switch elbows as needed. Sink in slowly. Vector down toward the client's feet.

Move in place (with tissue) down–up–down–up. Move down the back to T2–T3.

Repeat 3–4 times or as needed.

Thumb-over-thumb press: Examine for TPs and other sore, knotty, and crunchy areas. Press and hold each point for 5–6 seconds. Cross-fiber friction.

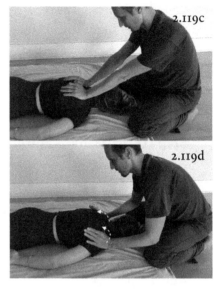

2.119c

2.119d

A: Double-palm press both sides. Hook into the **upper trapezius** or the spine of the scapula (**levator** and **supraspinatus**).

Press down toward the client's feet and hold for 7–8 seconds.

B: Lifting "cobra's hood"—hook your thumbs under the curl of the upper trapezius.

Press upward to "uncurl" the trapezius. Rock side to side. Change the position of your thumbs and repeat.

Repeat **Steps 109–119** on the other side.

After completing both sides, go to the next step.

Step 120. Crosswise back press

Transition: High Tripod or **Lunge.**

Tools: Heels of the palms.

Focus: Releases myofascial tissue jams between intervertebral joints.

Caution: Do not aim to "adjust" the client's joints. Our focus as massage therapists is myofascial tissue release, not joint adjustments. That is the work of chiropractors and osteopaths. We must be clear about our abilities and the scope of practice. However, occasional unintentional adjustments (cracks) may occur, although we do not force them or aim to elicit them.

Technique: 1–2 palm presses. Each press takes 1 second. The second compression is a little stronger and deeper than the first. Hook the heel of your palm at the client's posterior iliac crest, pressing downward (to the client's feet). Place your other palm on the opposite side of their spine, pressing upward and away from the spine (**Diagram 36**).

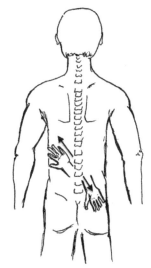

Diagram 36. Crosswise spinal joint traction

Perform the 1–2 palm press at the posterior iliac spine—both palms press at the same time in a 1–2 rhythm. Switch hands and perform the same technique on the other side of the iliac crest. Repeat two more times at the iliac crest, switching hands each time.

Move up along the spine to the upper back and stop at T2–T3.

Switch hands after every one or every two compressions.

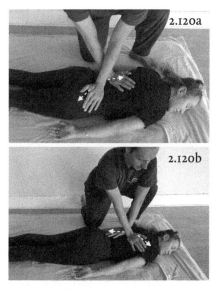

Step 121. Chop the back

Chop quickly both sides of the spinal muscles, from the glutes to the trapezius.

"Chopping" the muscles at the end of a treatment "informs" the muscles to tone up and return to a normal slightly toned state. This practice helps to "set" the muscles and joints in the proper alignment so the body does not "slide back" into misalignment if the tissues are too relaxed after the treatment.

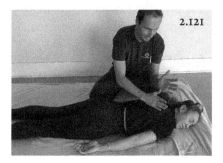

Prone—Pelvis and Legs

Step 122. Glute fist press and roll

Position: Tripod.

Sit across from the client's pelvis.

Fist press and fist roll over the glutes and hip external rotators.

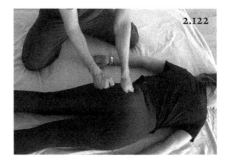

2.122

Step 123. Knee flexion

Pick up the client's foot. Press *over* the toes to push the heel to the buttocks: 1–2–3, mild–medium–deep.

Hold the deep flexion.

Fist press into the **glutes** at the same time.

Caution: Do not press too deeply. Many people have a limited range of motion in their knee joint due to prior ACL, MCL, and meniscus injuries. Always check in with clients.

Applications: Relaxes the glutes; stretches the hip flexors and psoas.

Variation: Knee press. Place your upper knee onto the client's **gluteus maximus**.

Press down on the client's foot and compress their pelvis (over the gluteus maximus) with your knee.

Perform 5–6 press–release compressions.

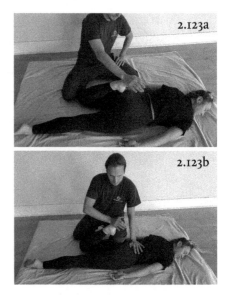

2.123a

2.123b

Step 124. Ankle dorsiflexion

Position: Tripod, or **Archer**, using your *knee as support* for their ankle.

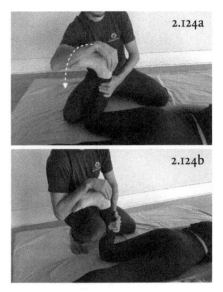

2.124a

Cup the client's heel with your lower hand.

Place your forearm over the client's foot.

Drop your elbow to "crank" the ankle.

1–2–3, mild–medium–deep.

2.124b

"Crank down and flex"—bring the client's heel closer to the buttocks, 1–2–3.

Variation: Achilles strip. Here is yet another way of working on the Achilles tendon and perhaps coming back for a short treatment of Achilles tendinitis (see **Clinical focus #2**).

Grasp over the Achilles tendon with your thumb and fingers.

"Flex and strip"—squeeze the Achilles tendon as you flex the knee and ankle.

Step 125. Ankle lift and shake

Position: Archer (as above), or **Tripod**.

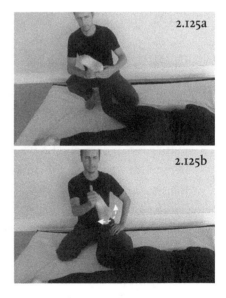

2.125a

Grasp the client's ankle with your thumbs and fingers. Lift and shake it a few times.

Hold over the toes and shake the heel and calves.

Hold the heel and shake the toes.

2.125b

Soft fist-pound over the bottom of the foot and heel.

Step 126. Hip rotation with glute press

Holding the client's ankle, move their leg in and out—away and toward you—external and internal hip rotation.

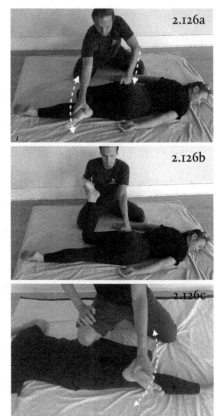

2.126a

2.126b

2.126c

Keep the gluteal compressions with your fist as you explore the gentle limits of their range of motion.

Circle their hips in both directions.

Repeat 8–10 times, switching the angles of pressure.

Variation: Knee press on glutes.

Transition: Archer.

Place your upper knee onto the client's gluteus maximus. Hold their ankle and rotate the hip.

Increase knee pressure gradually if comfortable for the client.

CLINICAL FOCUS #13: THE PIRIFORMIS

The piriformis is an external hip rotator. It also helps other muscles like the gluteus medius and gluteus maximus in pelvic stability. Contrary to popular belief, the piriformis is not a tight but generally weak and chronically overstretched muscle. To understand how a weak muscle becomes "tight" and the mechanism behind its weakness and seeming tension, see **Article 3** (on the **piriformis**) in the Appendix.

Occasionally, a chronically tight piriformis presses on the sciatic nerve that runs underneath. This condition is known as piriformis syndrome and is often mistaken for sciatica (see **Diagram 37**).

Clinical application: To release a cramped piriformis and to free up scar tissue from the overstretched muscle fibers.

"Pin and stretch" technique: Contract the piriformis by bringing the leg into external hip rotation (Photo C.13).

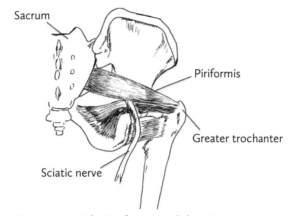

Diagram 37. The Piriformis and the sciatic nerve

Compress the piriformis at its greater trochanter attachment with your thumb or knuckles.

Rotate the client's leg into internal rotation—bring it in toward you—while holding the compression. Repeat compressions along the length of the muscle.

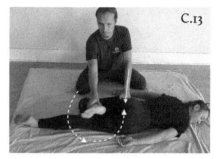

Add hip circles with compressions. The hip circles are performed in the TUAD direction (T—toward you, U—up, A—away from you, D—down).

TP and cross-fiber techniques: Holding the client's ankle, move their leg into external and internal hip rotation, looking for taut, tight bands within the piriformis tissues. Once located, press and hold for 8–10 seconds on each compression. Address points near the attachments.

Cross-fiber and with-fiber friction along the length of the muscle and its attachments.

Make sure to repeat on the other side.

CLINICAL FOCUS #14: SACRAL LIGAMENTS —"SACRAL MANDALA"

The sacrum is at the core of our stability, especially the stability of our spinal column. The sacrum itself is a stable structure. Its five vertebrae—S1 to S5—are fused naturally.

The sacrum is part of the axial skeleton. It articulates with the appendicular skeleton (of the lower body) at the bilateral sacroiliac joints via strong ligaments that allow only a minimal degree of movement.

When the strength of these sacral ligaments is compromised, the sacrum loses its stability, which leads to overall instability of the body, compensatory patterns up and down the chain, and potential injuries.

In general, ligaments are not elastic. They are not supposed to be stretched. Their job is to stabilize the joints they connect (see **Diagram 38**).

- If torn (from a fall or another injury), ligaments heal by developing scar tissue or adhesions that may limit mobility of the joints and restrict blood flow.

- If loose (from over-stretching), the joints lose stability and are more prone to injury.

In short, it's best to keep your ligaments strong and not stretched, and your muscles both strong and well stretched.

Sacral pain tends to be low, often on one side, extending into the buttock, the back of the thigh, and even the calf muscle. It may start suddenly and persist as a dull ache or a feeling of "pins and needles" in the butt.

Curiously, the age with the highest incidence of back pain is the same age at which the greatest mobility in the sacroiliac joints is available: 25 to 45 years old. This proves that greater mobility causes instability and leads to injuries.

Sacral ligaments are common sites of injuries and over-stretching. There are many things that may hurt (and overstretch) our sacral ligaments: pregnancy, sitting too much, not warming up before exercise, overstretching, playing contact sports, etc. It is very common to have adhesions, fascial restrictions, and pain around these ligaments.

Cross-fiber friction aims to "unstrap" those thickened and knotted bands of tissue. I call the following treatment **"Sacral Mandala"** because of the circular pattern of the release techniques applied. Not all of these tissues are ligaments. Some of them are familiar muscles we have already treated in previous clinical focus applications (**Diagram 38**).

Here is the pattern found in **Diagram 38**:

1. Iliolumbar ligament

2. Sacroiliac ligaments

3. Gluteus maximus attachments on sacrum and gluteal plateau

4. Gluteus medius and its greater trochanter attachments

5. Deep six external hip rotators, and their attachments on the femur and ischium

6. Gluteus maximus attachment on the femur (gluteal tuberosity)

7. Ischial tuberosity (hamstrings attachment)

8. Sacrotuberous ligament.

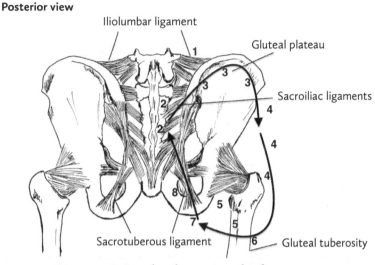

Diagram 38. Sacral and posterior pelvic ligaments

Position: Hero, Sit-and-Lean, or Spiral.

Sit right against the client's hip. Change your position as needed.

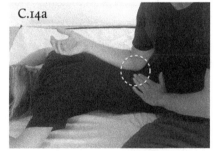

Use your inside elbow—elbow edge and elbow point—as your tools.

Elbow press or pulse into the iliolumbar ligament. Use your other hand to palpate for the right spot.

Caution: Do not hit the vertebrae. Press or pulse 4–5 times.

Hold and friction in place for 8–10 seconds.

Move your elbow down to the sacroiliac ligaments. Press or pulse 4–5 times along the length of the sacrum. Cross-fiber friction up-and-down over the ligaments.

Elbow press right off the sacrum to treat the gluteus maximus attachments. Cross-fiber friction in place up–down. Move out to the gluteal plateau. Elbow circle under and around the posterior iliac crest (Photo C.14b).

Elbow press and circle into the gluteus medius. For deeper pressure, connect your fist in your hand, and lock your elbow against your knee.

Cross-fiber friction at the posterior greater trochanter attachments of the gluteus medius and piriformis.

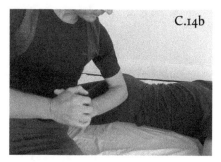
C.14b

Cross-fiber friction with your elbow on the deep six hip rotators. Treat their attachments—inferior to the greater trochanter on the femur and on the ischium.

Press and hold at the gluteal tuberosity—attachment of the gluteus maximus. Cross-fiber friction right against the femur.

Press and hold under the ischial tuberosity—right across the hamstrings. Swing your legs out to sit more comfortably (Photo C.14c).

Press or pulse into the sacrotuberous ligament (it feels like a bone). Draw an imaginary line between the client's ischial tuberosity and tail-bone (coccyx)—this spot will be in the center of this line. Cross-fiber friction in place.

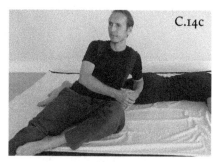
C.14c

Return up to the sacrum. Forearm circle around the sacrum with broad circles to "make nice."

Repeat the "Sacral Mandala" if necessary.

Step 127. Posterior ITB press

Position: Tripod or Lunge.

Keep the client's leg in internal hip rotation. Palm press down the posterior gluteus medius and ITB.

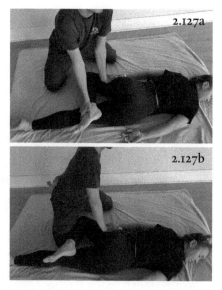
2.127a

Repeat 2–3 times.

Variation: Sacrum press with leg lock. Lock the client's leg with your lower knee.

2.127b

Palm press around the sacrum and the gluteal attachments.

Step 128. "Water pump" ITB press

Position: Tripod or Lunge.

From **Step 127** above, bend the client's straight leg to pin their ankle in the knee crease.

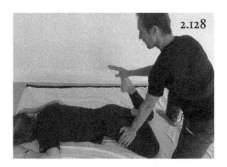

2.128

"Water pump" their foot, pressing heel to buttock.

At the same time, palm press down the ITB. Repeat for 2–3 rounds.

Caution: Do not press too hard, especially if the client has a history of knee injuries.

Step 129. Leg pull and shake

Transition: Squat, Hero, or Tripod.

Move down to the client's feet.

Hold the client's foot with one hand under and the other hand over.

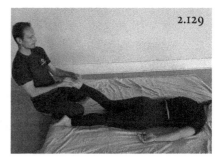

2.129

Techniques:

A: Pull–release, bouncing the leg off the floor.

B: "Toss" the foot hand to hand.

C: Shake the foot vigorously with one hand.

Step 130. Leg lift with sacrum foot press

Position: Hold the same ankle (as above) and stand up between the client's knees.

Turn 45 degrees in the same direction as the ankle you are holding (i.e., if you are holding the client's right foot, turn to the right).

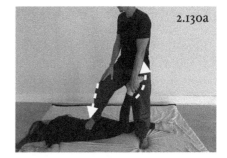

2.130a

Place your inside foot (left foot in the example above) over the client's sacrum. Your medial arch goes directly across the sacrum.

Caution: Do not step on the tailbone or lumbar vertebrae.

Make sure to grasp firmly around the client's ankle. Use both hands if needed to hold the ankle.

"Press, pull, and release"—step on with 50 percent of your weight and lift the client's leg. Hold for 1 second. Take your weight off your foot, releasing the client's leg down. Reposition your foot and repeat 8–10 times.

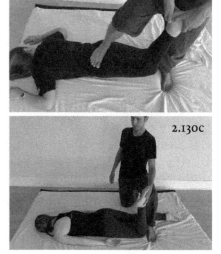

2.130b

2.130c

Use your heel to press around the sacrum, sacroiliac ligaments, and muscle attachments.

Avoid pressing directly on the sciatic nerve.

Lift and hold for 5–6 seconds on the last lift up.

Transition out of **Step 130** into **Lunge** on the other side.

From the standing position above, step your working foot (off of the client's sacrum) straight back behind the client's straight leg.

Bring your knee to the floor on the client's other side.

Optional: Repeat **Steps 123–130** on the other side before continuing to **Step 131**.

Step 131. Foot compressions on back (optional)

This is an optional technique that can be performed at this time or earlier, after **Step 107** ("back elbow compressions").

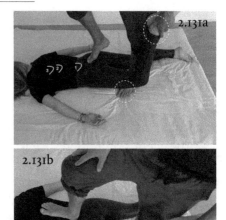

2.131a

2.131b

Before kneeling down after **Step 130**, continue foot compressions up the back.

Important: Do not pull up on the client's leg too high. Hold on to their ankle *only for your own balance*.

Use your heel.

Compress into these three specific locations, as shown in Photo 2.131a:

- Iliolumbar ligament

- Mid-back, around T8–T10 (under the "bra line")

- Mid-back, around T4–T6 (on the "bra line," between the scapulae).

Perform 2–3 rounds of compressions.

Caution: Do not press on the vertebrae or the floating ribs.

Perform **Step 131** on the other side.

Step 132. Supported hip extension

From the Transition after Step 130: Wrap your lower arm around the client's lower leg and grasp over their knee.

Place your upper hand on their sacrum.

"Press and lift"—palm press the sacrum and lower back. Reposition your compressions and repeat 8–10 times.

Press your front foot down to help lift the leg.

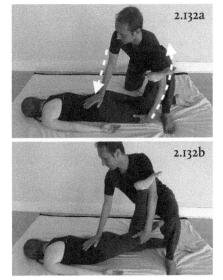

2.132a

2.132b

Step 133. Leg prop and press

Transition and positioning: Cross-Legged or **One-Leg-Out.**

From above, lean on the floor on the other side of the client with your upper hand.

Lift their knee with your lower hand and slide your upper knee under the client's thigh as far as the anterior iliac bone.

Straighten the client's leg and support it (prop it up) with your thighs, either in Cross-Legged or in One-Leg-Out position, whichever feels more natural.

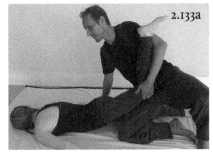

2.133a

Forearm roll up the **hamstrings**.

Elbow press and hold the **ischial tuberosity** attachments.

Elbow roll into the **gluteus maximus**.

Forearm roll the calves with your lower arm, if comfortable.

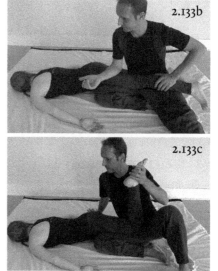

Transition out: Lift the client's ankle to 90 degrees. Hold the ankle with your lower hand.

Lean on your upper hand on the opposite side of the client (Photo 2.133c).

Pull the client's ankle straight up and lift their knee off the floor. Slide back out and bring your knee on the floor on the other side of the client.

Optional: Repeat **Steps 132–133** on the other side.

Prone—Additional Techniques

Step 134. Wheelbarrow

Transition: to **Standing.**

Holding the same ankle as in **Step 133**, pick up the other ankle and stand up between the client's knees.

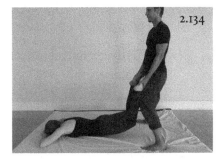

Bend your knees and keep your back straight before lifting the client's legs.

Step your feet shoulder-width apart and sway side to side gently.

Application: Provides relief to the lower back; mildly stretches the hip flexors.

Step 135. Bear walk

Setup: Hold the client's ankles and separate the client's knees to shoulder-width.

Step your left foot across the middle of the client's left hamstrings.

Hook the client's left foot in front of your left knee (Photo 2.135a).

Place your left hand over the client's sacrum and lean in.

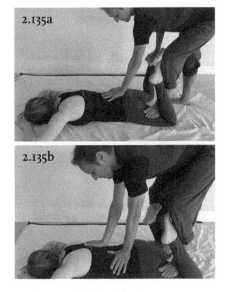

Using the three points of balance (left foot, left hand, and right hand holding the client's right ankle), step your right foot over the middle of the client's right hamstrings, and hook their foot in front of your knee.

Keep your knees bent. Palm walk up and down the back 3–4 times.

Transition out: Unhook the right ankle and step down with your right foot.

Unhook the left ankle and step down with your left foot.

Step 136. Cobra

Caution: Confirm the client has no low back pain or recent rotator cuff injuries.

Position: With your feet either on the inside or outside of the client's knees, kneel in the center of the gluteus maximus.

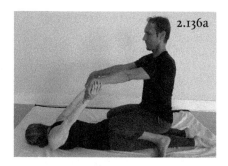

2.136a

Arm extension check: Take hold of the client's wrists and pull their arms into extension slowly.

Listen for their natural resistance—do not pull past it.

Rock from side to side, pulling on the client's arms.

Check if it is comfortable to lift the client's shoulders off the mat.

Note: Before lifting, tell the client *what* you are going to do. Have them grasp your wrists as well—this will help tremendously!

Suggested instructions: "Please bring your arms alongside and hold my wrists. I am going to lift you up slowly."

Use your body weight—lean back to lift them up.

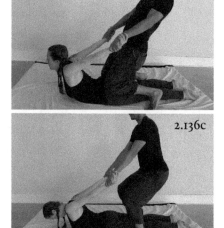

2.136b

2.136c

"Lift your chin gently and take a breath… Now, let your head hang and relax."

Hold for 2–3 breaths and release.

When releasing, tell the client: "Turn your head to either side and relax!"

Brush your hands over the shoulders and back to "make nice."

A. Standing. For tall and long-armed clients, stand next to the client's hips.

Pick up their wrists. Keep your knees bent, back and arms straight.

Lift very slowly, sensing how far is comfortable for the client.

Hold for 3–4 breaths.

B. Sitting. For better shoulder support.

Place a pillow on the client's sacrum.

Step your feet to the client's armpits.

Sit on the client's sacrum on the pillow (not on the lower back or tailbone).

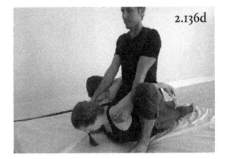

2.136d

Grasp each wrist, one at a time, and place it over your knee and at your hip.

Reach *under* the client's shoulder joints (acromioclavicular joints) and lift their upper girdle by leaning back.

Use your weight. Hold for 3–4 breaths.

Step 137. Child's Pose

Tell the client to push up and sit back on their heels with their arms forward (Child's Pose).

Position: Lunge. Lunge behind the client.

Palm press the back—sacrum to shoulders—2–3 times.

Grasp and squeeze over the upper trapezius.

If you are lightweight, kneeling gently on the client's sacrum may feel comfortable.

Variation: Back and shoulder traction.

Transition: Standing Lunge. Face the client.

Walk around and place your back heel between the client's hands.

Have the client clasp their hands firmly over your heel.

Palm press, pushing down to traction the back away from the shoulders.

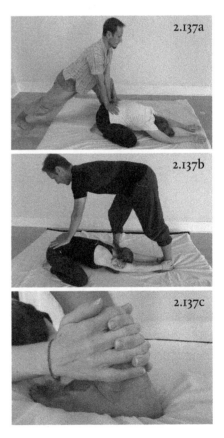

2.137a

2.137b

2.137c

Move your heel back—1 inch at a time—without losing the client's grip.

Repeat 3–4 times while pressing down at the client's ribcage, or the posterior iliac crest.

Transition: Ask the client to turn over onto their back (supine).

Side-Lying—Lower Body

Step 138. Supine twist

Position: Tripod.

Client in supine. Pick up the client's leg, bend it at the knee, and push the knee across into the twist.

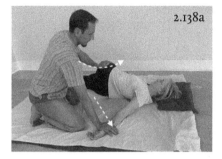
2.138a

Prevent the client from turning over to side-lying right away—catch their arm and keep it out-stretched. Press at their wrist.

Push at the posterior greater trochanter.

Rock them into the twist.

Rock in a slow rhythm, alternating between hip press and arm or shoulder press, for 10–15 seconds.

Transition: After the twist, pick up the client's wrist and bring their arm forward, in front of their shoulder.

Proper alignment:

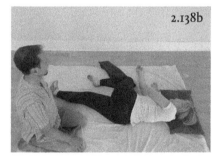
2.138b

- Client's top leg is bent at 90 degrees.

- Client's bottom leg is straight.

- Client's bottom arm is not pinched too close to their body; if it is, pick it up at the wrist and stretch it out.

Step 139. Foot and calf press

Position: Tabletop. Face the client's feet.

Knee press the client's medial arch with your inside knee.

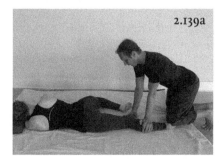
2.139a

Start with light pressure and stay away from the heel and toes.

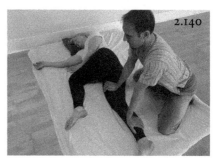

At the same time, palm press the calf with your outside palm.

Lean on your inside hand.

8–10 compressions.

Step 140. Bottom leg press

Transition: Tripod.

Move to the side of the client's straight leg.

Press in–press out.

Press into the **adductors** with your upper palm. Turn out your lower palm—point fingers toward you—and press the calf muscles away from the tibia.

Cover the length of the **adductors** and **calves**, 2–3 times.

Step 141. Blood stop on femoral artery

This is an alternative technique to **Step 13**.

Caution: Perform this only if the client is familiar with the "blood stop" technique. Blood stop blocks and "promotes" (after the release) the flow of blood in the femoral artery and related tissues (**Diagram 11**). It is important to ask before performing it. Discuss the benefits (below).

Contraindications: Pregnancy, high blood pressure, varicose veins, advanced osteoporosis, diabetes. Check with the client beforehand!

Good for: Circulation problems, edema in the legs, neuralgia in the legs, low back pain.

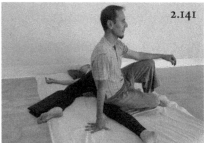

Transition: Sit-and-Lean.

Turn away from the client's leg. Face down and away from their head.

Lean on your arm, hover over the client's upper adductors, and place your weight slowly and gradually—use the center of your buttock.

Press and hold. Stay for 45–60 seconds.

Acknowledge the benefits of the technique with the client and check in on how they feel.

Release slowly. Repeat 2–3 times—more distally and more proximally to the initial compression—if needed.

Step 142. Leg press and roll

Position: Tabletop to **Lunge** and back.

Change positions to be more comfortable. Step over the client's leg if needed.

Techniques:

A. Palm press the client's top leg: shin, thigh, and hip.

B. Knee press on the adductors at the same time.

C and D. Forearm press the gluteus medius and roll the ITB.

Circle around the greater trochanter.

Supinate your forearm (start with your palm up, press down, and turn your palm down).

Roll down the ITB at different angles:

- Between the ITB and hamstrings
- Between the ITB and vastus lateralis.

Roll down 2–3 times.

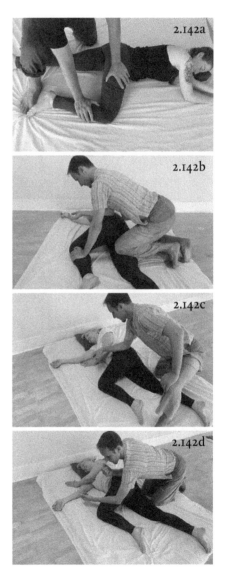

2.142a

2.142b

2.142c

2.142d

Step 143. Paddleboat

Transition: Step over the client's straight leg.

Sit and stretch your legs out. Place your feet on the client's hamstrings.

Grasp and pull at their ankle and walk your feet side to side, as in supine "paddleboat."

2–3 rounds from knee to hip.

Variation: Thigh press.

Positioning: Scoot in closer, bend your knees, and hook the client's foot over both of your knees.

Hook your fingers over the client's thigh and pull back.

Finger walk across the thigh (over the **quadriceps**) while pressing your feet into the client's thigh.

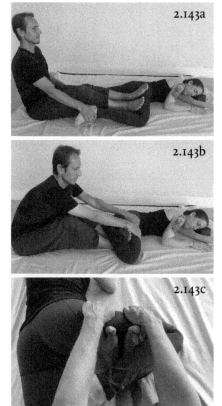

2.143a

2.143b

2.143c

Step 144. Hip muscles press and roll

Transition: Return to **Tripod** behind the client's hips.

A. Forearm and elbow. Make wide circles around the greater trochanter: gluteus medius and gluteus maximus, piriformis and other deep external hip rotators.

B. Elbow circle (deep circles) at the **gluteus medius** and **gluteus maximus** attachments at the greater trochanter.

C. Knee press and roll.

Transition: bring your upper knee to **Archer**.

Place your upper knee on top of the **gluteus medius**.

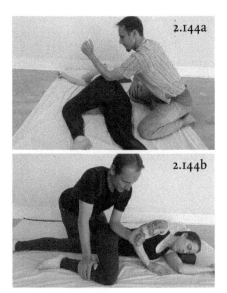

2.144a

2.144b

Reach over and place your upper hand on the floor and your other hand on the client's shin.

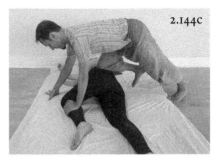

2.144c

Straighten your bottom leg.

Lift your foot for more pressure.

Rock forward and back—forward for more pressure, back for less pressure.

Important notes:

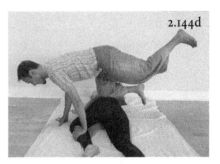

2.144d

1. Make sure to press directly on top of the gluteus medius.

2. Control the amount of weight by distributing your weight between your hands, knee, and back foot.

3. If more pressure is welcome, you may lift your back leg off the floor.

4. 5–6 compressions. Roll, or press, and hold steady.

CLINICAL FOCUS #15: PIRIFORMIS AND DEEP EXTERNAL HIP ROTATORS (THE "DEEP SIX") AND SACRAL LIGAMENTS

Side-lying is a great position for addressing these two areas as the hip is naturally exposed and easy to access.

A. In addition to treating the piriformis in prone (**Clinical focus #13**), it is important to address the other five external hip rotators: **gemellus superior and inferior, obturator externus,** and **quadratus femoris** (see **Diagram 39**).

Often, the pain and tension that clients complain about and mistakenly blame on their piriformis is, in fact, in one of the other deep rotators. Over-stretching (as in yoga) and over-working the glutes may cause cramping and micro-tears in these deep muscles. Often, these muscles harbor trigger points that feel extremely sensitive even with little pressure.

It is important to note that piriformis is the most superior, the largest and thickest of them, and the only one attaching at the sacrum and the femur. The other five muscles attach on the ischium and the femur.

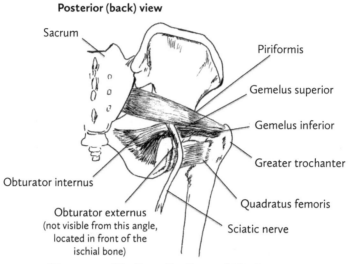

Posterior (back) view

Sacrum

Piriformis

Gemelus superior

Gemelus inferior

Greater trochanter

Obturator internus

Quadratus femoris

Obturator externus
(not visible from this angle,
located in front of the
ischial bone)

Sciatic nerve

Diagram 39. The Deep Six: External Hip Rotators

Position: Tripod.

Double-thumb press and thumb strip (Photo C.15 and **Diagram 40**); cross-fiber and with-fiber friction on the muscles in the following order:

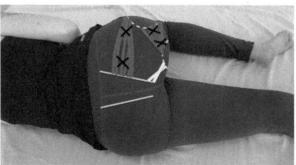

- **Piriformis** (most superior)

- **Gemelus superior**

- **Obturator internus**

- **Gemelus inferior**

- **Quadratus femoris.**

Obturator externus is not accessible from this angle.

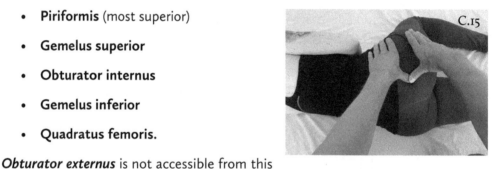

Diagram 40. Treatment points on the piriformis and other external hip rotators

Look for taut, tight bands and nodules. Hold "hot spots" and TPs as needed.

B. Treat the following ligaments: sacrotuberous, sacroiliac, sacrospinous.

Refer to **Diagram 41** below—similar to **Clinical focus #14** on the "**Sacral Mandala**."

Treat each of these ligaments to soften and "unstrap" any bunched up, fibrous tissues.

Thumb-strip. Cross-fiber friction. Hold "hot spot" compressions.

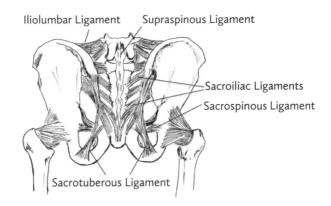

Diagram 41 Posterior Sacral Ligaments

Step 145. Quadratus lumborum scoop

Transition: Lunge.

Step up with your upper leg.

Muscles: Quadratus lumborum, obliques, transversus abdominis.

Scoop the tissue off the iliac crest with your thumb and the *web of your palm* (thumb down).

Rock forward and back as you press–release.

Double-thumb press for deeper compressions.

Press into the iliolumbar ligament 5–6 times.

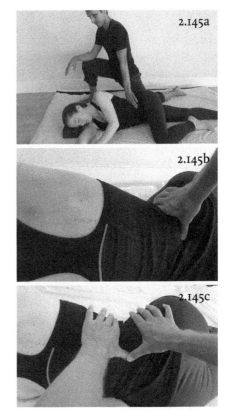

OPTIONAL CLINICAL FOCUS: LOWER BACK PAIN (DUE TO A TORN OR PULLED MUSCLE)

Refer to **Clinical focus #11** in **prone** and apply the same techniques: thumb-stripping, cross-fiber friction, and examining for TPs.

Side-lying position provides a higher angle of access to the multifidi and rotatores and may be more effective than the prone position (same as Photos 2.145b and 2.145c above).

Step 146. Back palm press

Transition: Tripod facing the client's back.

Palm press along the top half of the back, from the pelvis to the shoulder.

2–3 rounds.

It is possible to do the "thumb-chasing-thumb" technique on back lines in this position; if the prone position is not used or skipped due to neck injuries or discomfort, you may perform the back lines here.

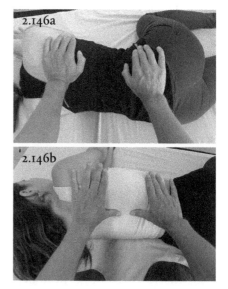

Step 147. Shoulder circles and trapezius lift

Place your hands over the shoulder girdle and circle 5–6 times in each direction.

Grasp and squeeze over the upper trapezius to warm up the muscles.

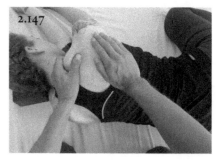

Step 148. Back elbow press

Transition: Sit-and-Lean, or **One-Leg-Out.**

Sit next to the client, hip to hip.

Turn 45 degrees away from the client.

Use your inside elbow for compressions—connect your hands and lock your outside elbow against your upraised knee for added weight.

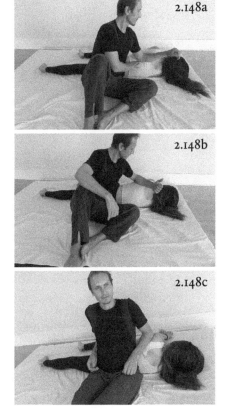

2.148a

2.148b

2.148c

Sink and hold compressions. Or sink and move your elbow in place (with tissue)—up-down–up–down 5–6 times.

Avoid hitting the spine. Stay in the lamina groove.

Move up the back, 1 inch at a time, from the sacrum to T2–T4. Repeat if needed.

A. Latissimus and ribs. Forearm roll over the latissimus and serratus anterior.

B. Latissimus and glutes.

Transition: Legs-Out.

Sit with your back against the client's back.

Place your forearms on the latissimus and glutes. Rock side to side 8–10 times.

Step 149. Arm extension

Position: Turn and stretch your legs alongside the client's back.

Reach over and take hold of the client's wrist. Bring their arm back into a comfortable extension.

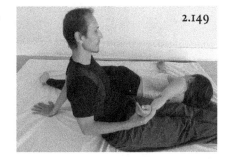

2.149

Lean back on your outside arm as needed.

Sense for the natural resistance in the ROM. Do not pull hard.

Hold the extension for 10–15 seconds.

Step 150. Shoulder pull

Drape the client's arm at your outside hip.

Grasp your hands over the client's shoulder (**upper trapezius**).

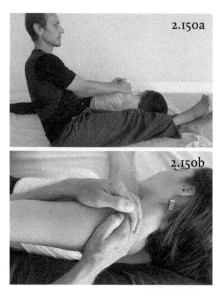

2.150a

Pull gently for 2–3 seconds and release. Lean your body back to pull.

Repeat 3–4 times.

Caution: Do not pull too hard (see **Article 4** in the Appendix for why shoulders should not be stretched deeply).

2.150b

Step 151. Upper trapezius and scalenes thumb glide

Setup: Cup the front of the client's shoulder with your inside hand.

Optional: Place the client's hand behind their hip (in the "arm lock" position).

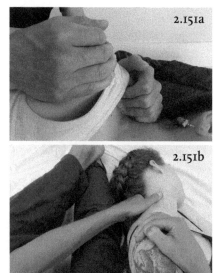

2.151a

Grasp and squeeze the **upper trapezius** with your outside hand.

"Pull and squeeze" (pull on the shoulder, squeeze on the trapezius).

Glide your thumb up the side of the neck. Pull back on the shoulder at the same time.

2.151b

Target each of the **scalenes**.

Glide along the **levator scapula**—from the "crunchy spot" on the superior angle of the scapula up to the transverse processes.

Glide all the way up to the **suboccipitals**.

Step 152. Arm extension push and pull

Transition: One-Leg-Out.

From **Step 151**, bring your hands out from the client's shoulder. Keep their wrist in your upper hand. Slide back and stretch your *lower* leg out.

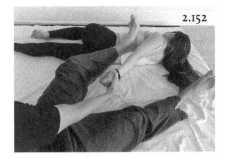

Place your foot on the upper half of the client's back near the **quadratus lumborum**.

"Push and pull" to elicit "joint play"—press your foot and pull on the arm.

Press along the lamina groove with your heel or ball of the foot. Press into the ribcage with your medial arch.

Important caution: Do not yank on the client's arm. Hold it for gentle extension only.

Note: The client's body must rock back and forth if this technique is done correctly. This move is to create a fluid rhythm of rocking, thereby releasing tension from the client's skeletal structure and spinal joints and eliciting "joint play."

Step 153. Latissimus compressions

Setup: Switch your legs.

Pull back on the client's shoulder until the client is almost halfway supine. This ensures that their arm will "hang by itself."

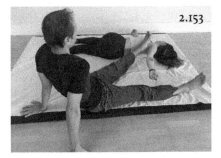

Technique: Rotate their arm out, thumb up.

Connect to the **latissimus** (on the lateral edge of the scapula by the armpit) with your heel or the lateral edge of your foot.

Press and hold for 8–10 seconds, letting the arm hang. Reposition higher *and* lower and repeat.

Step 154. Deltoid forearm roll

Transition C: Tripod.

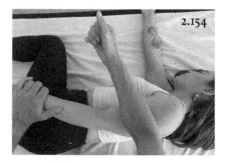

Hold the client's wrist down to their hip with your lower hand.

Forearm roll (supinate) along the **middle deltoid**.

Repeat 2–3 rounds.

Step 155. Scapula knee press

Transition: Archer.

Lift your upper knee.

Hold the client's wrist with your lower hand.

Hook your fingers over the front of the client's shoulder.

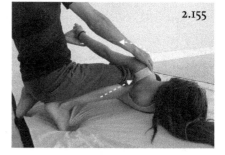

Pull back on their shoulder and knee press into the scapula (**infraspinatus** and **rhomboids**) with your knee.

To create compressions with your knee, plantar flex your ankle against the floor—press up from the ball of the foot.

Press all around the scapula—move your knee around, 8–10 compressions.

Pull back and hold for a couple of breaths to open the chest and reverse the mid-back "C-curve" (see **Article 5** on **mid-back pain** in the Appendix).

Step 156. Shoulder cradle with "arm lock"

Transition: Low Tripod behind the client's shoulders.

Setup: Place the client's arm behind their hip ("arm lock").

Slide your lower hand under the client's elbow and cup the front of their shoulder.

Technique: "Pull and push"—pull back on the shoulder and press your thumb or fingers into the **rhomboids** along the medial border of the scapula.

Press all the way to the **levator scapula** attachment at the superior angle.

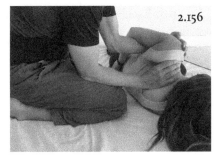

2.156

You may also use knuckles for compressions.

Brace your elbow against your upper knee for deeper compressions.

Perform 2–3 rounds along the scapula.

Step 157. Pectoralis treatment

Technique A: "Pin and stretch."

Transition: Lunge.

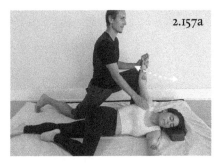

2.157a

Step up with your upper leg.

Setup: Hold the client's wrist. Circle their arm forward and up.

Bring their wrist across your upraised knee, switching hands.

"Pin and stretch"—grasp the bundle of pectoral muscles.

Squeeze between your thumb and fingers without poking. Use your fingerpads.

Stretch the client's arm out at different angles.

Look for tight spots and knots on the pectoral muscles.

Hold down compressions at **pectoralis minor**'s ribs 3, 4, 5 attachments (**Diagram 42**).

Add arm circles while holding compressions.

Technique B: Elbow press.

Transition: One-Leg-Out.

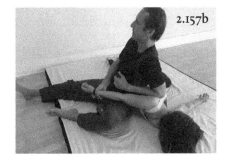

2.157b

Sit next to the client with your thigh against their upper back. Turn away from their back, with your outside leg out.

Line up your forearm with the client's upper arm. Sink in slowly with your elbow into the **pectoralis major** and its attachment on the humerus.

Lean back—your elbow will hit the spot!

Shift the elbow medially (closer to sternum) to hit the **pectoralis minor** tendon at the coracoid process and its rib attachments.

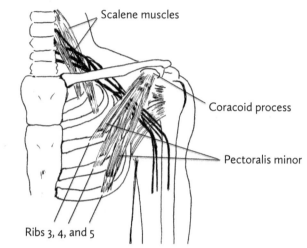

Scalene muscles

Coracoid process

Pectoralis minor

Ribs 3, 4, and 5

Diagram 42. Anterior shoulder view – pectoralis minor

Step 158. Anterior deltoid elbow press

Position: Same as "B" above. Swing your legs alongside the client's back to support their shoulder with your inside knee.

Use the "flat of the elbow" (not the point).

Support the client's shoulder underneath with your outside hand.

Roll over the anterior deltoids by supinating your forearm, 3–4 times.

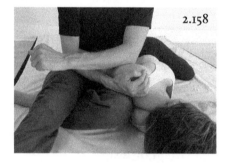

2.158

Step 159. Deltoid and rotator cuff grasping

Transition C: One-Leg-Out up to **Lunge.**

Lunge alongside the client's back. Hold the client's wrist with your lower hand.

Grasp over the client's shoulder joint—over the **deltoids**, **biceps tendon**, and the tendons of the **rotator cuff** muscles.

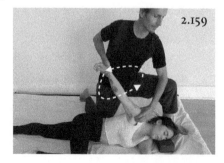

2.159

"Squeeze and rotate"—squeeze the shoulder between your thumb and fingers. Stretch and rotate the client's arm at different angles.

Be specific to the ropey or stringy tendons.

"Flick" your thumb or fingers over the tendons and muscles to "activate" them.

Cross-fiber friction a little longer to smooth out any thick nodules in the tendons.

Step 160. Lateral press and traction

Transition: Lunge.

Step up higher—place your foot over the client's head.

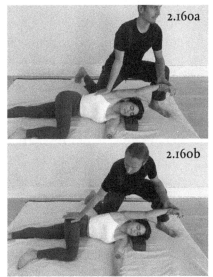

2.160a

2.160b

Switch your hands—hold the client's wrist with your upper hand.

A. Palm press down the client's side—over the scapula, ribcage, and down to the iliac crest.

Important note: Keep your fingers turned out, away from the client's breast.

B. Hook your palm over the iliac crest and traction from wrist to hip for 4–5 seconds.

Note: Make sure *not to slide* on the iliac bone to avoid "skin burn."

CLINICAL FOCUS #16: RIBCAGE CONNECTION—LATISSIMUS DORSI, SERRATUS ANTERIOR, AND INTERCOSTALS

Years ago, at a yoga therapy training, our teacher asked us to measure our ability to expand our ribcage during breathing exercises. We placed our hands on the front of our ribcage with our fingertips barely touching. A slow deep in-breath would expand the ribcage and draw the fingertips apart. A complete exhalation would contract the ribcage, bringing the fingertips back together, or even making them cross over. We were asked to work on our ribcage pliability to expand beyond 2 inches and possibly work up to 4 inches.

A tight and restricted ribcage may lead to a general sense of tightness around the chest, a feeling of suffocation and anxiety, asthma, breathlessness, as well as pain and chronic tension in all surrounding muscles. The **intercostals**, **anterior serratus**, and **latissimus** are the muscles critical to ribcage mobility and the feeling of ease.

The following techniques target these muscles. Some of the previous moves should be included with these techniques.

Ribcage release

Perform all the preceding steps of the above protocol, from **Step 152** to **Step 160**.

Transition: to **Tripod**. Scoop and grasp the tissue over the ribcage.

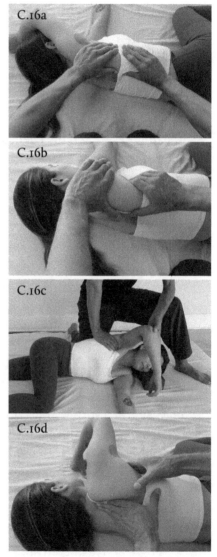

C.16a

Latissimus: Examine for TPs. "Lift" the **latissimus**—"sift through" and pull up—moving down from its insertion on the humerus along the lateral edge to the posterior iliac crest.

"Bone clean" the **latissimus'** origins on ribs 12, 11, 10, and 9.

C.16b

Serratus anterior: Place your hand over the client's ribs. Cross-fiber friction where your fingers fall—examine for TPs on each of the costal strip of the muscle, working from anterior attachments on ribs 9 to 3 back toward the edge of the latissimus.

Note: Keep the client's arm up to open the axilla.

C.16c

Serratus anterior: Slide your fingers over the ribcage toward the 1st rib (into the axilla)—compress down, examine for TPs (Photo C.16c).

Under the scapula: Place the client's fist on the mat and have them hold their arm in that position (Photo C.16d).

C.16d

Bring your inside hand anterior to the edge of the latissimus. Slide your outside hand under the medial border of the scapula.

Vector under the latissimus and as deeply into the space between the scapula and ribcage as possible, "hugging" the ribcage—examine for TPs.

Note: Give yourself enough room in front of the latissimus to get underneath them.

Grasp and jostle the scapula off the ribcage.

Intercostals: Transition back to Tripod. "Bone clean"—cross-fiber friction between the ribs into the **intercostals**. Double-thumb press on each individual rib to feel its firmness, responsiveness, and sensitivity to pressure. Press on each rib as if you are pushing it into its spinal joint (costovertebral joint).

Finish with palm circles to "make nice."

Step 161. Latissimus and triceps elbow press

Transition: One-Leg-Out.

Sit next to the client with your hip against their back.

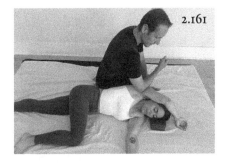

Keep your outside hand underneath the client's arm for support.

A hand towel may be used as a cushion between the client's arm and ear.

Use the "flat of the elbow" for compressions.

Go over the **latissimus**, the lateral border of scapula, and all the way up **triceps**.

Step 162. Chest opener nerve stretch

Transition: One-Leg-Out.

Scoot back and keep your *upper* leg extended.

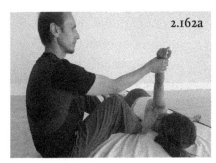

Place your foot on the client's scapula for support and to prevent the client from rolling back. Do not press on the scapula.

A. Hold the client's wrist. Raise their arm into the stretch very *very* slowly.

Find the "high angle," when the arm is stretched in the same direction as the fibers of **pectoralis major** (upward-sloping). This is the angle where the arm "hangs by itself."

Support under the wrist without pulling down—just let their arm hang.

B. Press down on the client's fingers. Uncurl them one by one, slowly, including the thumb, then all fingers at the same time.

Lighten up if too intense for the client—keep checking in with the client.

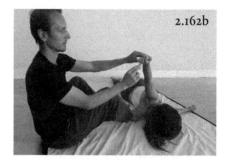

2.162b

Step 163. Under scapula toe press

Setup: Scoot in close enough to hold the client's shoulder.

Place the toes of your upper foot *under* the medial border of the scapula.

Note: Your toes are the tool, so keep your toenails trimmed! If working on skin, drape a hand towel over the client's shoulder.

Technique: Pull back on the shoulder with your upper hand. This will bring the scapula over your toes.

"Dive" your toes under the scapula.

Press your toes into the ribcage and "scoop out" tissue from under the scapula.

Repeat 4–5 times in the same spot.

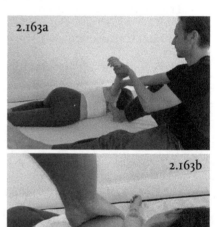

2.163a

2.163b

Reposition your foot up and down, all along the medial border.

I would also recommend keeping your toes on the **rhomboids** without much pressure—pull back gently on the shoulder and hold the client's mid-back in this open position, reversing the mid-back kyphosis, or the "C-curve" (see **Article 5** on treating **mid-back pain** in the Appendix).

Step 164. Foot walk on back

Foot walk on the client's back, holding their wrist with your upper hand.

Use your heels and balls of the feet.

Keep your upper foot at the mid- to upper-back/scapula area and your lower foot at the lower back and sacrum area.

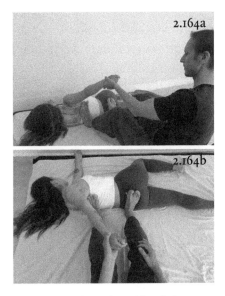

2.164a

Important note: The focus of this move is *not* pressure. It's rhythm!

The client's body should rock back and forth—eliciting "joint play"—back when you pull gently at their wrist while pressing with your lower foot, and forward when you release the wrist and press your upper foot.

2.164b

Avoid pressing directly on the spine.

Foot-walk along the back, 2–3 rounds.

Variation: Bottom leg pull. Lean over and take hold of the client's *ankle of the straight leg* (not the top leg).

Let the client bend their knee as far as comfortable for them.

Continue as above, while pulling on the leg and arm: Pull the leg, press the upper foot. Pull the arm, press the lower foot.

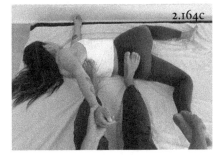

2.164c

Test to see how far is comfortable. If the client's hand and foot are able to touch easily, go to **Step 165**. Otherwise, bring their bottom leg back into the straight position and follow to **Step 166**.

Step 165. Bow Pose

(*For flexible folks.*)

Bring the client's hand and foot together and let them grasp their own ankle.

Keep your hands clasped over their hand and ankle to provide support.

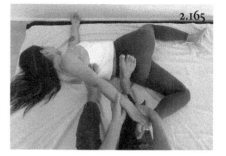

2.165

Hold the compression with your feet at their sacrum and mid-back for 8–10 seconds.

Important: Stabilize their sacrum with your bottom foot, to prevent their lumbar spine from arching. This is about hip extension!

Perform **Step 166** or **Step 167** (skip one or the other).

Step 166. Easy side-to-supine transition

Transition: to **Lunge**.

Grasp *under* the client's heel and *over* their knee with your hands.

Use your body weight to lift and roll them back into the supine position.

Do not drop their leg. Hold it at the heel. Straighten their leg by scooting down.

Give it a pull and a shake and let it go.

Repeat **Steps 138–166** or **Step 167** on the other side.

Step 167. Hip extension with glute compression

Transition: to **Lunge**.

Step your lower leg over the client's straight leg.

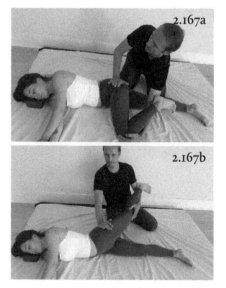

2.167a

2.167b

Setup: Slide your lower hand under the client's ankle and hold *under* their knee joint. Their lower leg should be resting on your forearm.

Place your upper hand on their hip/glute and keep their hips one above the other (to prevent them from rolling back).

Scoot back and pull their leg into extension. Push and pull 4–5 times.

Variation: Glute knee press.

Transition: to **Archer.**

Lift your upper knee and place it on their glute. Pull and press.

Pull the extended leg back—you can now hold it with both hands.

Press with your knee by plantar flexing from the ball of the foot (keep their hips aligned).

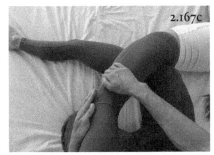

2.167c

4–5 times. Hold the last one for 8–10 seconds.

Transition out: Holding the client's leg, knee walk down and roll them onto their back. Give their leg a pull and a shake and drop it to the floor.

Repeat **Steps 138–167** on the other side.

Supine—Back Lifts and Stretches

Step 168. Lower back lift

Setup: Holding the client's ankles, stand up and lift the client's legs.

Walk up and place the client's heels on your hips or abdomen.

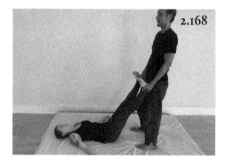

2.168

Rock your body back and forth—rock back and pull back—taking the weight off the client's lower back.

If comfortable, the client's lower back may be lifted off the floor and rocked side to side.

Step 169. Happy Baby Pose

Setup: Bend the client's knees by pushing them with your knees.

Keep their knees and feet apart.

Place your knees on the client's **hamstrings**, keeping your toes curled under and your thighs aligned at 90 degrees down.

"Pin and stretch"—move your hands on to the client's heels. Lean in forward with your knees, pressing straight downward, and push the client's legs up.

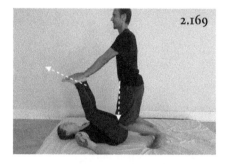

2.169

Important: Keep the angle of your thighs at 90 degrees (straight down). Otherwise, the "bent knee" position puts too much load on your knee joints.

Reposition your knees, closer to the ischial tuberosities. Repeat 5–6 times.

Hold the last compression for 8–10 seconds.

Step 170. Double hamstring stretch, aka "speedskater"

Setup: Step over the client's legs and push your calves against the client's thighs, locking their legs into the straight position.

Important: Do not push back too hard.

Rock leg to leg, gently turning your body side to side and pulling on the client's legs.

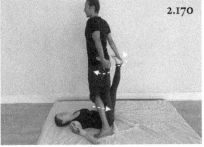

Step 171. Bound Angle Pose

(*For flexible clients only.*)

Step your feet up under the client's armpits, still holding the client's legs.

Most people will bend their knees at this point. If they do not, give their legs a shake to bend the knees, or ask your client to bend their knees.

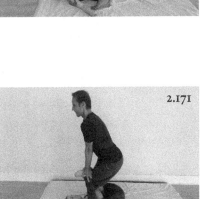

Slowly bring the soles of the client's feet together in front of your thighs and press their feet toward their face.

Keep your back straight, lock your elbows, and bend your knees.

Press 1–2–3, mild–medium–deep.

Step 172. Shoulder Stand

(*For flexible clients only—with healthy necks.*)

Setup: Keep the client's feet together.

Ask the client to firmly place their hands on their thighs and lock their elbows.

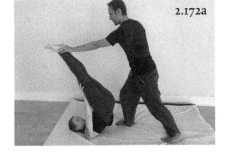

Technique: Step your feet into a wide walking stance. Push the client's legs up directly toward their head, lifting their body off the mat *until their hips are directly above their shoulders.*

At this point, their body will stay in this position more easily.

Caution: Do not push up past this point—that could strain their neck!

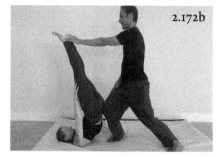

Support their weight with your knee against their sacrum. This will take some pressure off their neck muscles.

Hold for 8–10 seconds.

Step 173. Supported Bridge Pose

Caution: This is an advanced technique *for practitioners*. Perform only if you are strong and flexible in your hips and knee joints and have strong legs and core muscles. Practice first with a friend who is lighter than you.

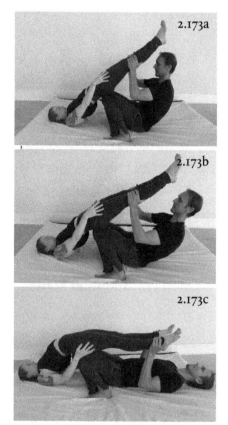

A. From Shoulder Stand above, place your knees on the gluteal plateaus (superior to the gluteus maximus bellies) off the sacrum.

Keep your knees together while your feet are shoulder-width apart, with your hips in internal rotation.

Slowly lower the client's legs to your shoulders and, if comfortable for the client, down to your hips.

Sit back on your heels.

You may pause here and hold for 8–10 seconds before lifting back up.

B. If comfortable with "A," hold onto the client's hips and roll onto your back very slowly.

Rest on your back for 15–20 seconds.

To lift up, walk your hands up to the client's knees or thighs. Hold them at the sides and pull yourself up.

Step 174. Lift up transition

A. Cross-legged lift—not recommended. This is a classic transition, pulling people up from supine to seated.

The client's ankles are crossed and rested against your knees. You hold the client's wrists and pull them up to seated. However, I have seen this move cause back pain and shoulder tension. It may also cause discomfort in the knees for older and inflexible clients and would be contraindicated for anyone with osteoporosis. In short, it is safer to avoid this move. Instead, perform "B."

B. Arm-pull transition to seated. This is a much safer way to bring clients into the seated position.

Step over the client. Take hold of their wrists.

Rock side to side and gently traction the client's arms.

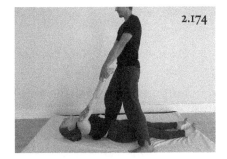

2.174

Tell your client that you'd be lifting them to be seated. Most people will automatically "help you" when they know what to expect.

Walk your feet back as you pull the client up to **seated forward bend**. Rest their hands on their legs.

Seated—Back, Neck, and Shoulders

Step 175. Forward bend back press

Transition: Lunge.

Walk around the client's back and step down.

Push the client into a comfortable forward bend.

Squeeze their shoulders.

Palm walk down the back, 2–3 rounds.

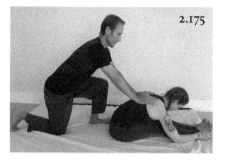

2.175

Step 176. Top of shoulders palm press

Position: Stand up and pull the client up by their shoulders.

Tell them to cross their legs.

Support the client's back with your front knee, or with both knees. It helps to angle (turn) your front foot inward.

Palm press straight into the client's shoulders.

Press 8–10 times from different angles: close to the neck, and farther from the neck.

Caution: Do not press too hard so not to overstretch shoulder muscles (see **Article 4** on **shoulder stretching** in the Appendix).

Muscles: Upper trapezius, levator scapula, splenius capitis and cervicis, scalenes.

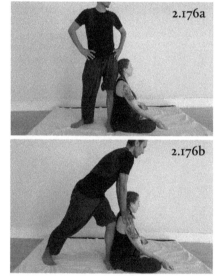

2.176a

2.176b

Step 177. Trapezius press and roll

Transition: Lunge.

Step down to Lunge.

Support the client's back with the inside of your upraised knee.

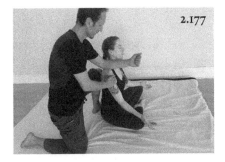
2.177

Use your inside elbow to press and roll (i.e., supinate) into the top of the shoulder (**upper trapezius**, **levator scapula**, **supraspinatus**).

Support the client's shoulder with your outside hand.

Grasp and squeeze the upper trapezius with your outside hand while pressing and rolling into the muscles.

Note: Refer to **Article 4** in the Appendix for details on **neck and shoulder muscles**.

Step 178. Shoulder ROM

Hold the client's wrist and move their arm in different ways:

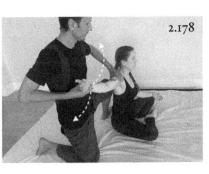
2.178

- Lift up into full flexion. Pull back into extension. Open up into abduction.

- Circle around in each direction, 2–3 times.

Finish by tucking the client's hand behind the lower back, as in Photo 2.179a.

Step 179. Scapula pop, in arm lock

Position: Archer.

Use your knee to pin the client's wrist to their back.

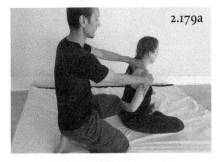
2.179a

Caution: Do not pull the client's hand high up. Just leave it low behind their hip or lower back.

Technique: Pull back on the client's shoulder with your outside hand.

Thumb press the tissue off the medial border of the scapula all along the edge.

Use knuckles as an alternative tool.

Lean in with your elbow into the **rhomboids** and **levator scapula**, if comfortable.

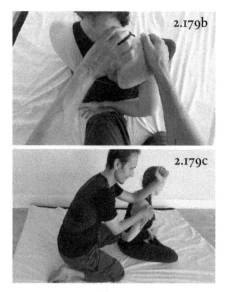

Step 180. Water pump

Transition: Lunge.

Setup: Bring your inside knee away from the client's back. Rest your inside elbow on your knee and place your hand on the client's back for support.

Pick up the client's wrist (with the outside hand, i.e., your right hand picks up their right wrist). Switch your hand position on the client's wrist so that your elbow points in and up, and your thumb points downward.

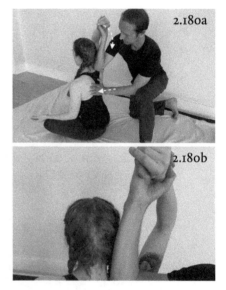

Technique: Place your elbow directly on top of the client's shoulder.

"Crank the water pump"—pull the client's wrist toward the midline. This will drive your elbow deeper into their shoulder. Reposition and repeat 8–10 times.

Target the levator scapula attachment and upper trapezius.

Finish: Bring the client's hand into their lap.

Repeat **Steps 177–180** on the other shoulder.

Transition: Lunge to **Lunge**—knee down/knee up.

Bring your upraised knee down. Step your other knee up on the other side of the client.

Step 181. Scalp and temples circles

Stand behind the client and support their back with your knees.

Place your fingers on their temples and your thumbs on their scalp above the hairline.

Circle your fingers on the temples 8–10 times. Circle your thumbs on the scalp 8–10 times.

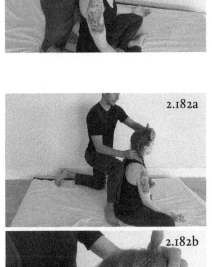

2.181

Step 182. Neck/scalenes circles

Transition: to **Lunge.**

Use the inside of your upraised knee to support the client's back. Place your outside hand on the client's forehead to support their head.

Wrap your fingers and thumb around the back of the client's neck.

Thumb press and thumb circle along the **scalenes** in up–down strips from posterior to anterior. Finger circle on the opposite side at the same time.

2–3 strips from posterior to anterior.

2.182a

2.182b

Step 183. Occipital press and decompression

Support the client's forehead, as above.

Squeeze the **suboccipitals** between your thumb and fingers. Tilt the client's head back at the same time.

Move your compressions all along the occiput.

Cervical decompression: Tilt the client's head back and lift. Repeat 5–6 times.

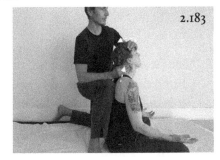

2.183

Transition: Lunge to **Lunge**—knee down/knee up.

Bring your upraised knee down. Step your other knee up on the other side of the client.

Repeat **Steps 182–183** on the other side.

Step 184. Cross-legged forward bend

Push the client forward into forward bend.

Note: Tell your client what to do so they do not resist you.

Squeeze over their shoulders.

Palm walk down the back and the thighs, 2–3 rounds.

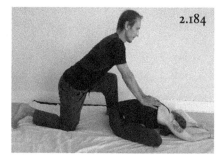

2.184

Step 185. Arm-pull back traction

Setup: Stand behind the client. Support the center of their back with your front leg. Angle (turn) your front foot inward, same as in **Step 176**.

Ask the client to interlace their fingers over their head.

"Thread" your front arm under the client's interlaced hands. Cup your other hand over their fingers.

Step back to pull them up. Rock forward to release. Repeat 4–5 times.

Your feet should be a walking distance apart, in the "Tai Chi stance."

Variation (for tall and long-armed people): Bring the client's wrists together, fingers together (not interlaced).

Press their wrists together and rock back and forth, as above.

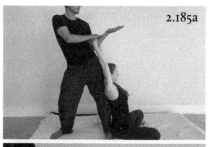

2.185a

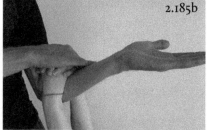

2.185b

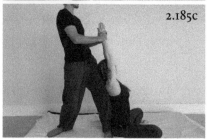

2.185c

Step 186. Chest opener

Position: Lunge.

Bring the client's interlaced hands behind their head.

Place your knee between the scapulae without putting any pressure on the spine.

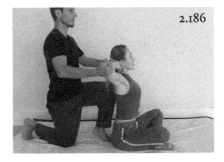

2.186

Hold under the client's elbows and gently pull back.

Mild–medium–deep. Hold on "deep" for 5–6 seconds.

Variation (for sensitive (bony) spine and knee): Stand up and place both of your knees on the client's mid-upper-back.

Repeat the technique in this position.

Step 187. Seated spinal twist

Position: same as in **Step 186.**

Rotate the client, pivoting around your knee.

Gentle–medium–deep to one side.

Switch sides.

If your knee is too pointy, or the client's spine is too bony, use both knees in the standing position.

Variation: Threading through the arms. This variation allows for better control of the client's shoulders and for a deeper twist; however, it is more difficult to perform.

Position: Archer.

Setup: Scoot in closer to the client. Place your upraised knee over the client's thigh *without* pressing on their thigh.

"Thread" your hands under the client's arms and hook your fingers over their forearms.

Technique: Push forward, lift, and twist. Push the client's body forward, lift them back up toward you, and twist them away from your upraised knee.

Rocking 1–2–3, mild–medium–deep. Switch sides—perform the same technique on the other side.

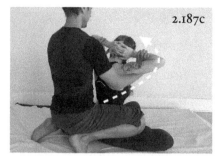

2.187c

Step 188. Seated lateral stretch

Face the client's side. Place the client's hand over their ear. Ask them to hold it.

Hold on to their opposite wrist.

Technique: Press the client's lifted elbow and pull on their wrist at the same time.

1—pull gently; 2—deeper; 3—even deeper. Hold for 2 seconds. Switch sides.

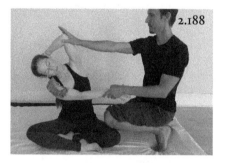

2.188

Step 189. Foot walk on back

Position: sit behind the client.

Hold the client's wrists.

Walk your feet on their back gently.

Dig your toes under the scapulae.

Rotate the client's arms out and pull back.

Perform 2–3 rounds up and down the back.

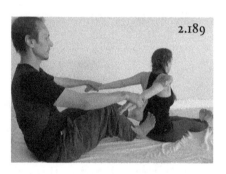

2.189

Step 190. Supported lumbar arch

Note: You will need a pillow.

Setup: From **Step 189**, rest the balls of your feet on the client's posterior iliac crest (your heels must stay on the mat). Curl your toes back. There should be about 1 inch of space between your big toes.

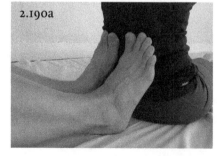

2.190a

Keep your knees bent (inch up closer, if needed).

Place a long pillow over your knees.

Ask the client to recline over the pillow— their head should rest between your knees.

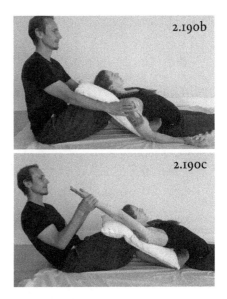

2.190b

Hang out here for 10–30 seconds.

Variation: Arm pull. Ask the client to raise their arms. Take hold of their wrists and pull back to traction their back and shoulders.

At the same time, press your feet into their iliac crest.

2.190c

Variation: Advanced (*for flexible lumbar spines*). Press your feet into the client's iliac crest. Slowly straighten your knees. You may recline all the way back, if comfortable. Rest here for 10–30 seconds.

Transition out: Bring the client's arms back to the front. Push your hands *into the pillow* at the level of the client's neck and shoulders and push them up to a seated position.

Supine—Neck

Step 191. Neck cradle and ROM

Transition: Wide Angle Pose.

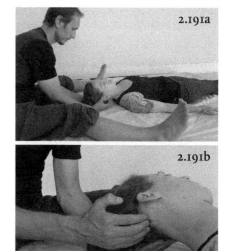
2.191a

2.191b

From **Step 190**, scoot back and separate your legs. Ask the client to roll back.

Catch their head in your hands before they get to the floor.

Cradle their head and place your fingers on the occipital ridge.

Rotate their head left and right.

Tilt the head, ear to shoulder, in each direction.

Lift and lower the head in a wave-like motion, 4–5 times.

Step 192. Neck lines

Cradle the client's head in one hand. *Do not* cover their ear. Rest your hand on the floor.

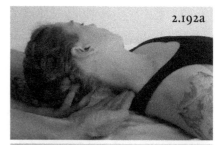
2.192a

Muscles: Cervical erector spinae, scalenes, levator scapula, splenius capitis and cervicis.

Line 1: With the fingerpads of your other hand (middle finger), locate the spinous processes of T1 or T2.

Circle next to the spinous processes up to the **suboccipitals**.

Repeat as needed.

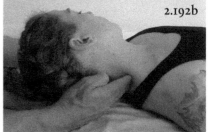
2.192b

See also **Clinical focus #18** on **neck pain** below.

Line 2: Repeat on line 2 (lamina groove)—press and circle.

Line 3: Bring your fingers under the client's neck. Stick out your thumb.

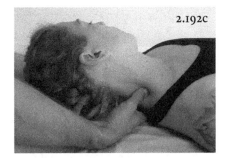

2.192c

Thumb circle and glide up/down line 3 (**posterior scalene**). Repeat as needed.

See also **Clinical focus #17** on the **scalenes** below.

Repeat the lines on the other side.

CLINICAL FOCUS #17: THE SCALENES

The scalenes are the three muscles found on each side of the neck, spanning between the transverse processes of C1–C7 and the upper two ribs. The main functions of these muscles are forward flexion, lateral flexion, and rotation of the neck. They also assist with respiration, elevating the ribs during forced inspiration.

Their position on the side of the neck places them in the delicate proximity to the busy pathways of spinal nerves and blood vessels. Chronically tight and short scalenes are known to entrap the nerves, causing thoracic outlet syndrome (see **Clinical focus #8** on the **brachial plexus**), restricted respiration, chronic neck tension and pain, and tension headaches.

Releasing the scalenes with Neuromuscular Therapy (NMT) can have immediate and profound benefits. It is possible to work on scalenes only in side-lying position, as in **Step 151**. However, it is advisable to treat scalenes twice, that is, return for **Round 2** in **supine** at the end of the treatment, as follows below.

Rotate the client's head and cradle it on one side, as in **Step 192** above. Thumb circle, or two-finger circle along the transverse processes from the mastoid process downward. Compress the transverse processes and thumb glide or "bone clean" in a superior to inferior direction.

Posterior scalene: Sink and melt just posterior to the transverse processes (not in the lamina groove) and move down. This is exactly the same technique as **line 3** in **Step 192** above.

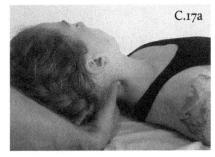

C.17a

Thumb press anterior to the edge of the upper trapezius and vector down *toward the 2nd rib*, the attachment site of the posterior scalene (see **Diagram 43**).

Cross-fiber friction on the spot.

Middle scalene: Sink and melt right into the transverse processes and move down. Search for TPs around the C3 area.

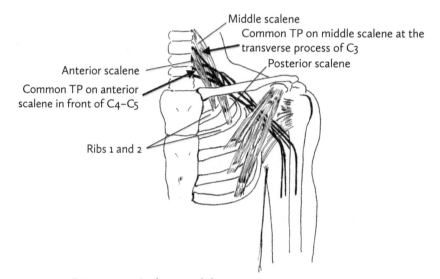

Diagram 43. Scalenes and their common trigger points

Anterior scalene: Compress into the anterior aspect of the transverse processes. Use your thumb or fingers to search for TPs. A common TP is at C4–C5 level (see **Diagram 43**).

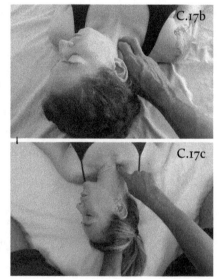

Gently "bone clean" the anterior aspect of the transverse processes with superior to inferior friction. Go down as close to the clavicle as possible.

Anterior scalene insertion on 1st rib:

- Lift and support the client's head at a 45-degree angle with one hand. Rotate the head away from the side being treated (Photo C.17c).

- With your other hand, compress your index or middle finger into the gap between the clavicular and sternal attachments of the sternocleidomastoid, vectoring toward the 1st rib attachment of the anterior scalene.

- As you lower the head, flex your fingertip and stroke up the belly of the anterior scalene. It's parallel to the sternocleidomastoid, and usually very tender. (Ask the client to lift their head—it becomes visible.)

"Make nice" by thumbing down gently on the side of the neck.

Repeat on the other side.

CLINICAL FOCUS #18: NECK PAIN

Chronically tight neck muscles may lead to restricted blood flow and painful muscle spasms, as well as postural distortion in the cervical vertebrae and spinal nerve impingement. There are many muscles that could become chronically tight: scalenes, splenius capitis and cervicis, suboccipitals, levator scapula, and upper trapezius, to name a few. We have already treated many of them in our protocol. In this section, we will focus on releasing the levator scapula, splenius capitis and cervicis, and suboccipital muscles. Additionally, see **Article 4** in the Appendix.

Levator scapula compression and release

Originating on the first four cervical vertebrae (C1–C4), this muscle extends down and inserts at the superior angle of the scapula (see **Diagram 44**). Its infamous "crunchy" spot at the superior angle indicates how often it gets strained and develops adhesions (that's what makes it so crunchy).

Place your fingerpads on the superior angle of the scapula.

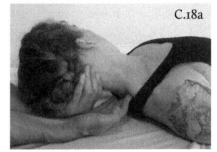

C.18a

Cross-fiber friction and finger circle on the attachment—smooth out the crunchiness.

"Pin and stretch"—press on it and roll the client's head to the opposite side. Repeat 2–3 times.

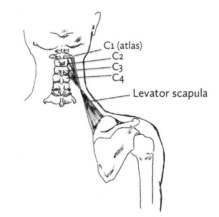

C1 (atlas)
C2
C3
C4

Levator scapula

Diagram 44. Levator scapula – posterior view

Splenius capitis and cervicis release

These deep muscles often escape the attention of therapists. Their proximal position and a powerful pull on the cervical spine and cranium make them likely culprits in neck tension and pain (see **Diagram 45**). The capitis inserts at the mastoid process, and the cervicis at the upper cervical vertebrae.

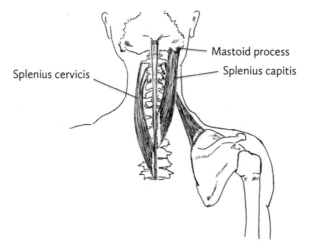

Diagram 45. Splenius capitis and cervicis

A. Slide your hand under the client's neck. Stick out your thumb.

Thumb press over the flap of the upper trapezius into the angle between the neck and shoulder.

Vector toward C7–T3 (origins of the splenius capitis).

Hold the compression and roll the client's head to the same side. Repeat 2–3 times. Cross-fiber friction in place.

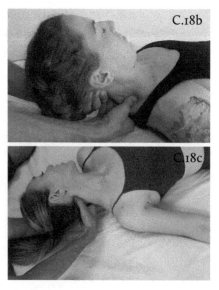

B. Slide your hand even deeper down the client's upper back. Stick your thumb out to T3–T5 (splenius cervicis). Cross-fiber friction against the spinous processes of T3–T5 and lower (as in line 1). Thumb press against the vertebrae and roll the client's head to the same side. Move up one vertebra at a time as you repeat the head roll until you reach C2 and C1.

C. Place your fingerpads on the posterior mastoid process (insertion of the splenius capitis) and "bone clean" gently side-to-side and up–down.

Suboccipitals

These overused "Yes" and "No" muscles shorten during computer use and chronic forward head posture, and become chronically tight and tender. They attach to C_1 and C_2, atlas and axis, and these two vertebrae are put under a lot of stress and considered the most important vertebrae in the health and alignment of the cervical spine (see **Diagram 46**).

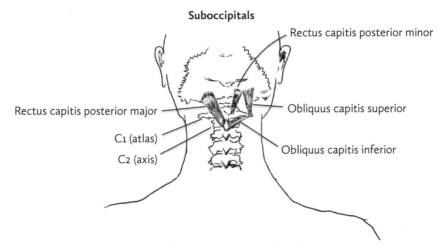

Diagram 46. Suboccipitals

Cradle the client's head in one hand and roll it away from the side being treated.

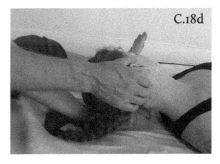

Hook your fingers under the occipital ridge and cross-fiber friction across and up–down—treating the medial to the lateral along the entire width of the occipital ridge to the mastoid process.

Repeat the same cross-fiber friction right on the occipital ridge. And once more, above (superior to) the occipital ridge.

Repeat on the other side.

CLINICAL FOCUS #19: WHIPLASH AND STERNOCLEIDOMASTOID (SCM)

Whiplash may occur when the head is thrown during an auto or sports accident. The neck is snapped back and forward (see **Diagram 47**). All neck and shoulder muscles are impacted. However, the muscle that bears the brunt of the trauma as it braces the head during the "snap" is the bilateral sternocleidomastoid (SCM).

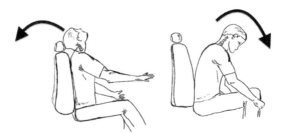

Diagram 47. Whiplash injury

Its name is indicative of its attachments: the sternum, the clavicle, and the mastoid process (see **Diagram 48**). It rotates the head to the opposite side when acting unilaterally, and flexes the head forward when both sides contract.

The forceful snap of the neck causes tiny muscle tears at the attachments and in the muscle bellies. Inflammation, scarring, and TPs follow. Many of these TPs are latent (not felt unless pressed). Nevertheless, they restrict movement and cause chronic tension, pain, and headaches.

Sternocleidomastoid (SCM)

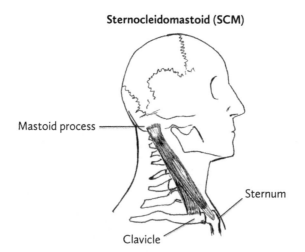

Diagram 48. Sternocleidomastoid

Pain patterns of SCM spread all over the head, neck, and face. How many different complaints turn up at the doctor's office that may, in fact, have their origins in TPs of the SCM? Headaches, neck aches, earaches, eye aches, toothaches, sinus aches, sore throats, even contributing to temporomandibular joint dysfunctions.

During the intake process, ask your client if they have ever had a car accident. They may have suffered a whiplash many years earlier and never realized that it had been precisely the cause of their ongoing *normal* neck pain and headaches.

Treating SCM requires a thorough understanding of its anatomy and a sensitive touch. The muscle lies superficially so it is both easily visible and palpable. However, the carotid pulse may be felt in the middle third of the front edge.

Under the SCM region runs a neurovascular bundle containing the carotid artery, the carotid sinus, the jugular vein, and the vagus nerve. These structures need to be avoided with direct pressure. The artery is the main blood supply for the brain. As long as you are not compressing these structures and not feeling any pulse under your fingertips, you and your client are okay.

When "picking up" the muscle with your fingers and thumb, it may be helpful to use a fine tissue paper (like Kleenex) so the muscle does not slip, especially if you or the client has oily skin.

Trigger points can be found throughout the SCM, both in the sternal and clavicular attachments and in the two muscle bellies. Some TPs lie in the deeply buried fibers of the clavicular head near the mastoid process.

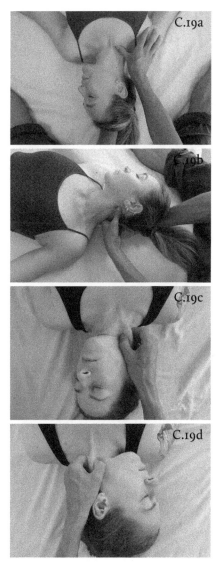

C.19a

C.19b

C.19c

C.19d

Techniques: Support the client's head with one hand (hold underneath or brace it at the side).

Rotate the client's head to the same side as your support hand.

Sternal and clavicular: With your thumb, "bone clean" the sternal and clavicular attachments—cross-fiber friction against the bones (Photo C.19a).

Mastoid: With your fingers (middle and index), find the mastoid process and finger circle against the bone. Perform a couple of deep compressions (Photo C.19b).

Muscle bellies: If the muscle is not visible, ask the client to lift their head—the SCM will "pop up."

Grasp it between your thumb and fingers. Use fine tissue paper if needed.

Roll the ropey muscle—examine for nodules and hold the TPs—between the thumb and fingers, working along the length of it, from the sternum to the mastoid.

Release and reposition lower and higher several times.

Repeat on the opposite side.

Step 193. Neck traction

Hold under the occiput with one hand.

Press over the client's shoulder with the other hand. Traction gently for 4–5 seconds.

Switch sides.

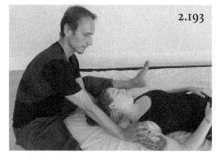

Step 194. Neck forearm roll

Hand position: Cradle the client's head in one hand.

Slide your other hand under their neck and place your fingers over the client's opposite shoulder.

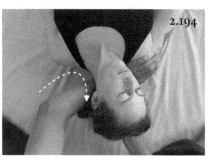

Technique: Roll your forearm into the client's neck. Your elbow makes a circle: away–up–in–down (away from you–upward into the client's neck–in toward you–elbow drops down).

Repeat 5–6 times.

Switch sides.

Step 195. Occipital ridge decompression

Muscles: Occipital attachments of the spinalis, suboccipitals.

Hook your fingertips under the occipital ridge.

Hold for 8–10 seconds.

Rock back and forth.

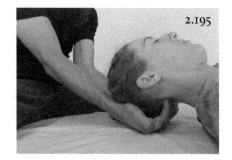

Hook your fingertips over the occipital ridge. Hold and rock, as above.

Face and Scalp

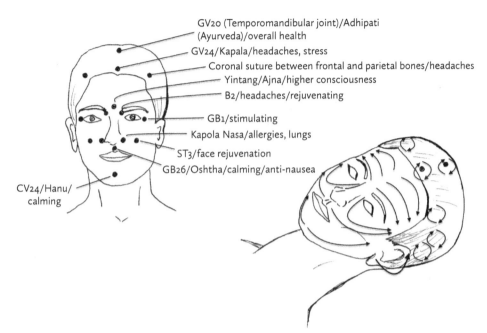

GV20 (Temporomandibular joint)/Adhipati (Ayurveda)/overall health
GV24/Kapala/headaches, stress
Coronal suture between frontal and parietal bones/headaches
Yintang/Ajna/higher consciousness
B2/headaches/rejuvenating
GB1/stimulating
Kapola Nasa/allergies, lungs
ST3/face rejuvenation
GB26/Oshtha/calming/anti-nausea
CV24/Hanu/calming

Diagram 49. Common points and lines

Step 196. Forehead thumb strokes

Rest your fingers on the sides of the client's head.

Strip your thumbs from the midline out to the temples in 3 or 4 lines (**Diagram 49**)—high (hairline), middle, and low (over eyebrows).

Repeat from top–down twice.

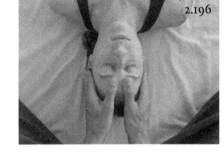

2.196

Step 197. Temple circles

Use your thumbs or fingers to circle at the temples.

Circle 3–4 times in one spot and reposition 3–4 times.

Step 198. "Open up" frontal bone

Place your fingers under the supraorbital ridge of the eye socket.

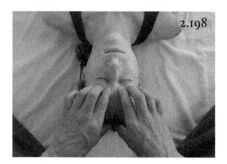

2.198

Index fingers go on B2 Bladder Point (see **Diagram 3** of **common acupoints**).

Place your thumbs above the hairline.

Hook the fingers and lift up—as if "opening a treasure box"—while pressing your thumbs down above the hairline.

Press–release a few times.

Step 199. Under eye socket press

Place your thumbs on the infraorbital ridge.

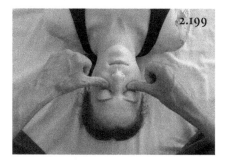

2.199

Press and hold for 3–4 seconds.

Repeat 3–4 times.

Caution: Avoid touching the eyeballs.

Step 200. Carving cheekbones

Use the fingerpads of the middle fingers.

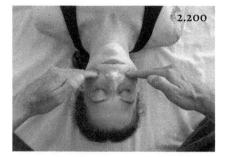

2.200

Start at the sides of the nose.

Press down and wait until the fingers melt into the tissue under the cheekbones.

Carve around and up toward the temples.

Repeat 3–4 times.

Caution: Avoid stretching the skin or causing "skin burn."

Step 201. Upper lip glide

Glide your thumbs out from the nose and up toward the temples.

Repeat twice.

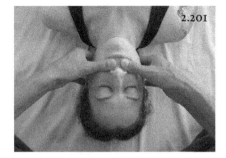

Step 202. Chin squeeze and glide

Squeeze the client's chin with your thumbs and fingers.

Slide out along the jawline toward the temples and circle on the **masseter**.

Repeat 2–3 times.

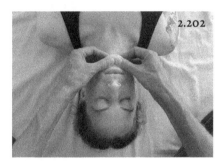

Step 203. Ear squeeze and pull

Hold the ears—thumbs on top, fingers under.

Squeeze gently and pull out lightly.

Move from the ear lobes up.

Caution: Do not pull hard on the ears.

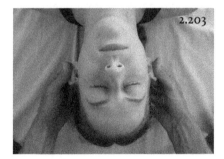

CLINICAL FOCUS #20: JAW PAIN AND TENSION AND THE TEMPOROMANDIBULAR JOINT (TMJ)

TMJ stands for temporomandibular joint and is the articulation point between the jawbone (mandible) and the skull (temporal bone) in front of the ears.

The following muscles are usually responsible for chronic jaw pain in the TMJ: masseter, temporalis, and the pterygoids (medial and lateral) (see **Diagram 50**). The pterygoids are mostly inaccessible from outside, unless intraoral treatment is performed, which is outside the focus of this book. However, both the temporalis and masseter are critical muscles in the jaw's healthy function.

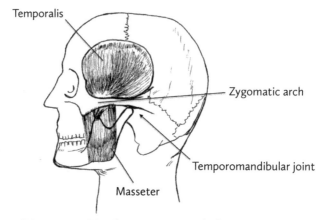

Diagram 50. Muscles causing TMJ dysfunction

Masseter release

Begin with carving around the cheekbones, as in **Step 200** above. Pause under the cheekbones and finger circle on the taut bands of the masseter.

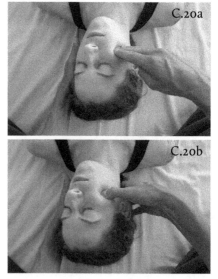

Tilt the client's head to one side and support it with the opposite hand.

Finger circle into the muscle tissue. Search for dense nodules or TPs.

Cross-fiber friction the attachments at the zygomatic arches (cheekbone).

Finger press up into the cheekbone—"bone clean" the attachments.

As an option, ask the client to open and close their jaw while holding tender points.

Then, use your thumb to glide downward away from the cheekbone, smoothing out the taut bands of the muscle.

Switch sides.

Temporalis treatment

Support the client's head on one side with your hand.

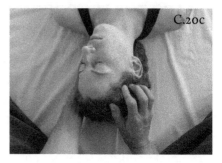

Hook the fingers of your other hand into the temporalis and circle in place.

Use flat palpation, looking for taut bands and nodules.

Press and hold the TPs for 8–10 seconds.

Cross-fiber friction gently. Look for dips and depressions.

Reposition—work from the ear up to the parietal sutures.

Caution: Do not scratch the scalp.

Switch sides.

Step 204. Scalp points and circles

Hook your fingers into the scalp above the ears. Place your thumbs on top or above the hairline.

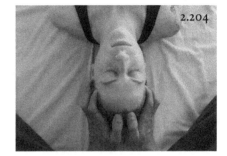

2.204

Circle and move the fascia of the scalp. Do not scratch.

Reposition, looking for depressions within the scalp, as well as sutures between the temporal, frontal, and parietal bones (see **Diagram 50**), and repeat 3–4 times.

Step 205. The finish: Third Eye circles, traction, and palm over

Glide your thumbs up the center of the forehead—from between the eyebrows to the hairline—3–4 times.

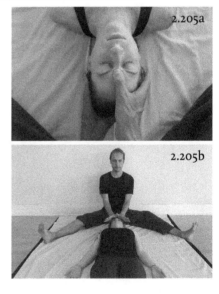

2.205a

2.205b

Use your thumb or middle finger to press and circle between the eyebrows (the Third Eye point)—wide circles leading to smaller and lighter circles. Then stop and hold for a few seconds.

Cup over the client's ears (without pressing on them). Hook your fingers into the occipital ridge and traction the neck gently for 8–10 seconds.

Hold your palms over the client's eyes, letting them feel the warmth and energy of your hands.

Appendix

Article 1: When to stretch the calf muscles

There are three muscle groups[1] that every runner should stretch on a regular basis. The calf muscles are one of these. If you are not a runner but are physically active, it is still a good idea to stretch the calf muscles once or twice a week. The only time *not* to stretch the calves is when they are pulled, torn, or otherwise injured.

The calves include the deeper-lying thicker soleus, and the more superficial double-headed gastrocnemius (**Diagram 51**). Both of these muscles merge into the Achilles tendon.

The Achilles tendon, as all other tendons in the body, is not elastic, meaning it is a set length, incapable of being stretched beyond its length. To stretch a tendon is to tear it. Hence, the only way to gain relief in the Achilles tendon from any tightness is to stretch its attaching muscles, the calves.

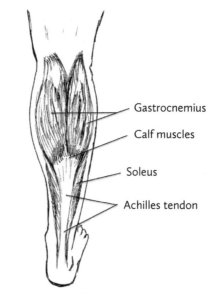

Diagram 51. Posterior lower leg muscles

---

1   The other two muscle groups are the hamstrings and hip flexors.

What if the calves suddenly feel tight?

This may be due to weakness in specific fibers within the calves. As we age, we lose muscle tone and muscle mass. If you experience sudden onset calf muscle tension, several fibers may have become too weak for your basic everyday load.

The best solution for getting rid of muscle tension is to strengthen the affected muscles.

Start with two sets of 15–20 repetitions of heel raises, or eccentric heel drops (see **Diagram 52**). After a week of daily sets, the tension will subside, or disappear altogether. To build more tensile strength and fiber density in the calves and the Achilles tendon, hold a dumbbell over your shoulder during the exercise.

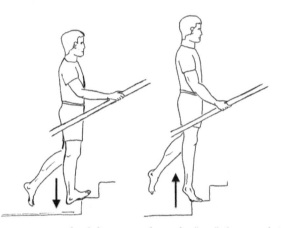

Diagram 52: Eccentric heel drops, quick on the "up," slow on the "down"

Why it is important for runners to stretch the calves

After a run, the calf muscles respond to the exercise by getting tighter. If not relaxed (being massaged, rolled, and stretched), they will remain tight, creating a strong continuous pull on the Achilles tendon. After the next run, the same thing happens. But now, an even stronger pull is being applied to the tendon. And so on, after each run. If not relaxed, at some point the Achilles tendon is not able to maintain its length and begins to tear and become inflamed (Achilles tendinitis).

Calf muscles can become tight even if you are not a runner. It is generally a good idea to stretch and massage them.

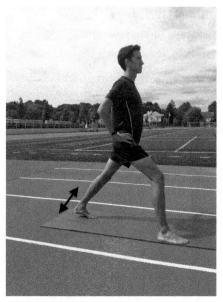

Professional runner, Timothy Ritchie, demonstrates dynamic calf stretches

The most effective way to stretch the calf muscles is to step one leg back, plant the heel on the floor, and hold the stretch for at least 1 minute. The long hold will create more length in the calves.

Holding for less time (10–30 seconds) will not be as effective to create permanent length, but is still beneficial to relax the muscles.

A straight-leg stretch targets the gastrocnemius muscles, while a bent-knee stretch targets the Soleus.

Please note—if you have a tear, or tendinitis, stretching is contraindicated as it will only deepen the tear or make the tendonitis worse. It's best to perform eccentric heel drops before performing any long-hold stretches.

General stretching rule of thumb: stretch only healthy tissue.

Article 2: The secret to resolving iliotibial band syndrome

If you've got a nagging pain on the outer part of your knee, especially if you're a runner, it could be a symptom of iliotibial band (ITB) syndrome. This is an injury often caused by activities where you bend your knee repeatedly, like running, cycling, hiking, and walking long distances.

The ITB is the longest tendon in the body. It originates out of a hip flexor muscle called the tensor fascia latae at the iliac crest (pelvic bone), and attaches down at the outside of the tibia (shin bone) (see **Diagram 53**).

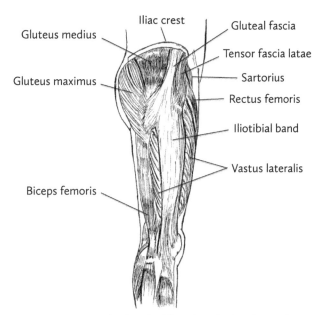

Gluteus medius
Iliac crest
Gluteal fascia
Tensor fascia latae
Gluteus maximus
Sartorius
Rectus femoris
Iliotibial band
Vastus lateralis
Biceps femoris

Diagram 53. The iliotibial band and related muscles

The ITB is extremely strong (stronger than steel in pound-for-pound tensile strength). Many people think the ITB is a muscle!

All tendons attach to muscles and form myofascial bundles that work together. Therefore it's not unreasonable to think the ITB is kind of like a muscle. However, there are a couple of very important differences:

- Muscles are more vascular than tendons (supplied with better blood flow), therefore tendons take longer to heal.

- Muscles are elastic = stretchy. Tendons are inelastic, meaning that tendons cannot be stretched without being torn or structurally compromised.

Unfortunately, ITB syndrome is a common condition that we often see in clients, especially in active people. Pain in the ITB can have several causes. The most typical cause is overloading the hip muscles with "too much too soon" activity such as a longer-than-usual run or hike, a long car trip or airplane travel, or a new activity that your muscles are just not used to. The response is tension in the hip muscles, resulting in a deep tightness in the ITB, and a painful, sharp or dull, sensation at the outside of the knee.

Does massage help?
Absolutely, but not because the ITB itself needs to be massaged. In fact, any massage on the ITB would be contraindicated during an acute episode of pain. However, massage will help to release hip muscles, thereby creating relief in the

ITB. The bordering hamstrings and quadriceps can be released as well, thereby "ungluing" the ITB from them and allowing it to move freely.

Fortunately, the pattern of the ITB pain is very similar in most cases. Usually, we get a call from a client that goes something like this:

> "I have this pain down my IT band. It's been going on for weeks. I am really disappointed because I have a race [or a ride] coming up next weekend, and I was really hoping it would be resolved by now."

> "How long has it been?" I ask.

> "Oh, it's been 3 or 4 weeks already." [Sometimes longer.]

> "What have you done to resolve it?"

> "I am stretching it every day. Foam-rolling religiously. Not exercising as much." [This is a typical response.]

> "Alright, you can stop stretching it," I usually say. "And you should not foam-roll an inflamed tendon either."

> "Why!?" They sound surprised. "My PT [or trainer] told me to roll it and stretch it."

> "For one, you cannot stretch the IT band," I explain. "It's a tendon, therefore it's inelastic. So by stretching it, you are only tearing at it and possibly causing more damage."

> "What should I do?"

> "Let's book a massage appointment. We'll work on the surrounding tissues and any tight muscles that might be the cause of it. And we will talk about a plan for faster recovery so you can still run your race."

I have had this conversation with hundreds of clients. The pattern of pain and tension tends to be very similar, as well as the cause of the ITB pain. In order to describe the cause, we cannot talk about the ITB without mentioning a pivotal muscle in the health of the hip and knee joints: the **gluteus medius**.

The gluteus medius

The gluteus medius is a pivotal muscle in the most literal sense—our pelvis is capable of pivoting on our femurs thanks to the gluteus medius (among other muscles). Its main job is to stabilize the head of the femur in the hip socket (**Diagram 54**).

The gluteus medius is designed for this complex stability work. However, in modern humans, this muscle has become the culprit of many, if not most, hip- and knee-related issues, including ITB syndrome.

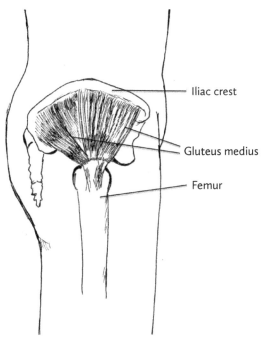

Diagram 54 The Gluteus Medius

In most people these days, the gluteus medius is too short and too weak.

Too short—because we sit too much. Too weak—because we don't know it exists—it's on the side of our body and we cannot see it in the mirror. Most people know about their quads and hip flexors, hamstrings and glutes, but mention the gluteus medius and people get a long look and point somewhere around their hip in a vague motion.

When the gluteus medius is too short and too weak, it is not capable of stabilizing the femur or the pelvis effectively. During a run, a ride, or another workout, the gluteus medius fatigues and stops working. Yet, your pelvis must be stabilized. You cannot be wobbly. Therefore, the gluteus medius *recruits* other muscles to assist it.

The most common muscle that comes to its assistance is the tensor fascia latae (the muscle of the ITB), since they are right next to each other and share fibers. Because the tensor fascia latae is not designed for stabilizing the hip, it promptly tightens up and pulls on its tendon. The person feels tension and pain along the ITB, especially at the lower attachment on the outside of the knee joint.

This is when people try to stretch and roll and massage their ITB. Does it work? Not really.

Chain reaction that leads to ITB syndrome
A weak and short gluteus medius leads to:

1. Instability in the hips and pelvis

2. The tensor fascia latae is recruited to help in stability, but

3. The tensor fascia latae is quickly overloaded and cramps or tightens up, and

4. The ITB is pulled tight and starts to ache and tear at the knee attachment.

How do we break this chain reaction?

By strengthening the heck out of the gluteus medius. Once the gluteus medius is strong, it will stop fatiguing during workouts. It will also stop recruiting the tensor fascia latae, and the pain in the ITB will go away on its own.

This recovery should take 5 to 7 days of performing a daily exercise that isolates the gluteus medius: side-lying leg lifts (**Diagram 55**).

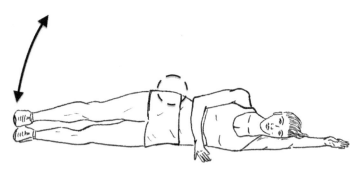

Diagram 55. Side-lying leg lifts

Lie down on your side. Make sure you are balanced. Lift your top leg 20 times. Perform two sets on each side with 1-minute rest in between sets. You may rotate the lifting leg upward and downward to emphasize anterior and posterior fibers respectively. Work up to two sets of 30.

In my opinion, this is the best exercise for the gluteus medius because the muscle is forced to fire during the side-lying leg lifts. There are other good exercises, such as clamshells and monster walks with a strap, but these exercises recruit other muscles. If the gluteus medius is used to "getting a free ride" by recruiting other muscles, it may do that during these exercises as well. I often call the side-lying leg lift "the Jane Fonda" because the exercise icon popularized this move in her aerobics videos.

Article 3: The scoop on the piriformis

The piriformis is a deep external hip rotator. It rotates the hip outward and stabilizes the pelvis, especially during movements such as walking and running, so we don't wobble (**Diagram 56**).

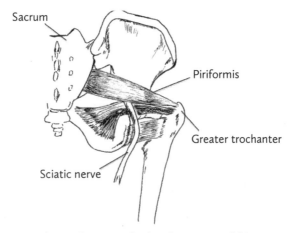

Diagram 56. The piriformis and other deep external hip rotators

The piriformis is one of those muscles that is rarely well understood by most people, including those in the healthcare field. For example, most people believe that their piriformis is too tight and must be stretched. As a result, there are many recommendations by yoga teachers, personal trainers, and even physical therapists to stretch the piriformis with such exercises as the Number 4 stretch, Pigeon Pose, and cross-legged forward bends.

Usually, such stretches provide temporary relief, while pain or tension doesn't get better in the long term. I do not recommend these exercises or stretching this muscle at all because they are not necessary!

What happens when the piriformis feels tight?
And does it actually get tight?
Yes, it does get tight, but not for the reason most people think.

There is a technique in massage called "pin and stretch." This is when we "pin" or compress a certain muscle and stretch it at the same time. This achieves a lengthening of the muscle fibers and a greater range of motion in the related joints. An example of "pin and stretch" is the pectoralis muscle stretch. We pin the pectoralis muscle against the ribcage and move the arm away at different angles. After this technique the shoulder enjoys a greater mobility and a rush of blood flow through the pectoralis.

"Pin and stretch" is also what we do to our butt and the piriformis when we sit down. We pin it to the seat (a car seat or office chair) and put our hips into forward flexion (sitting position). Often, we will deepen that stretch by crossing our legs or ankles. This means that your piriformis is being stretched quite a lot. In fact, in most people, the piriformis is overstretched.

What happens to a muscle that has been overstretched? Two things.

1. It becomes weak and loses its ability to perform its function well (in piriformis, it's stabilizing the pelvis).

2. It gets into a state of spasm (contraction).

The first one is clear—overstretched and weak muscles do not work very well. But how does a weak overstretched muscle go into a spasm?

Neural inhibition

When a muscle becomes stretched to its maximum length and held in that position for a long time (longer than a minute), it sends a signal to the brain: "Help! Release the stretch! I need to return to my neutral position to avoid tearing."

But it doesn't return to neutral because we continue to sit and stretch it. The brain forces it to contract, also known as a spasm or a cramp—a forced contraction to prevent tissue damage. And what do people do when they feel a spasm or a cramp? Well, they stretch it even more, of course.

We are told to stretch it. We believe it will relieve the spasm, as occasionally dynamic stretching does. But usually we hold deep piriformis stretches and cause tiny tears in the cramped muscle. Now it's weak, cramped, *and* torn!

When we sleep, the body (due to its innate intelligence) repairs the tiny tears. It lays a patch of collagen fibers. What happens when we wake up? We feel the repair work—the piriformis "feels" tight, because the body patched it up a little bit. Here is the clincher: *We mistake the sensation of tightening, healing, or patching up for tension.* We say: "My piriformis *feels* so tight. I keep stretching it and stretching it."

So we go ahead and hold those deep stretches again. Of course, we rip apart all that patchwork or repair work. We believe this kind of stretching "feels" like a good kind of pain—it feels like we are really pulling it apart, ripping it, because that is exactly what we are doing—ripping apart the healing bonds.

The next night the healing process repeats itself. And the next morning, we "feel" tight again, and so we stretch. And so on.

This can go on for months, never getting better. Slowly getting worse. Constant ache and inflammation develop. The cramping muscle may press over the sciatic nerve causing a painful nerve sensation in the butt and down the leg. Eventually, those microscopic tears become full-blown adhesions that we, massage therapists, are able to feel with our fingers.

What to do?

For starters, stop stretching your poor piriformis. Very few of us ever need to stretch that muscle. Strengthening the piriformis will support the healing process. In essence, it will support the body's efforts to repair it and tighten it back so it can function again.

At first, tightness means that healing bonds are forming. Don't rip them apart! Once the muscles get stronger, they will stop "feeling tight." They will relax and actually feel longer and healthier.

We are taught that tension is "bad" and flexibility is good. In reality, this is not the case. *Tension is good—in most cases, tension means strength and stability and efficient function.* Too much flexibility means possible instability, weakness, and loss of efficiency in movement.

Article 4: Should we stretch the trapezius and other neck muscles?

"I try to stretch my shoulders all the time, but it doesn't seem to work—they are just so tight!" This is what many people say when they arrive for a massage.

We are taught to stretch those tight muscles on top of the shoulders and the sides of the neck. These muscles include the upper trapezius, levator scapula, splenius capitis and cervicis, and the scalenes (**Diagram 57**).

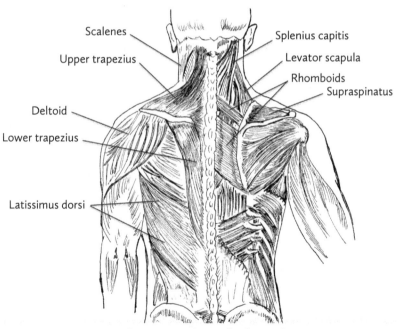

Diagram 57. Major back muscles

Well-meaning yoga teachers and exercise trainers tell us to do the ear-to-shoulder stretches—sometimes by pressing down on the side of the head to "deepen" the stretch. In fact, I've seen this very stretch promoted in a popular massage magazine.

We stretch these muscles, yet it doesn't seem to work. Why is that?

I believe it's not only *unnecessary* to stretch these muscles, but also *harmful* if you are trying to relieve tension there.

Let's take a closer look.

Each muscle has a certain range that it is comfortable with, as far as stretching and loading. Generally, the weaker the muscle, the smaller its range. For example, your upper trapezius is able to extend to a certain point until it begins to fight the extension, that is, resist the stretch, in order to protect itself. This is known as **neural inhibition**—our body's natural mechanism of protecting itself from damage—so we don't hurt ourselves when we don't pay attention.

Thanks to neural inhibition, our muscles contract when they are stretched beyond their end point. This way they will not tear. This makes sense, right?

However, we seem to ignore this basic concept when we stretch our neck and shoulders.

During the day, our upper trapezius, levators, and other muscles in the neck and shoulders are pulled down—they support our arms, which hang down most of the day. Whether we are driving, sitting at a computer or sitting down to eat, running or hiking, biking or taking a stroll, most of the time, these muscles are pulled down and basically stretched taut to their maximum end point.

After a while, a few hours of being stretched taut, all of these muscles start to contract to protect themselves from over-stretching and over-tearing. As they contract, they start to *feel* tight because the *sensation* of contracting is the *sensation* of tightening. Unfortunately, we misread this sensation for tension that needs to be stretched. So we force them back into their maximum stretched-out position. Finally, the muscles are not able to handle this over-stretching, and they tear—tiny microscopic tears that heal with collagen fibers.

The next day, this process repeats. The shoulder muscles are pulled down all day without relief, we misinterpret the sensation of over-protection for tension, and...we stretch them! And, of course, more microscopic tears occur. And again, and again.

Over time, this becomes a pattern; the built-up collagen, now a scar tissue, palpable and often visible, aka "the crunchy spot," aches and bothers us non-stop.

So let me pose the initial question one more time.

Do you think we need to stretch our neck and shoulders?

By now, the answer should be obvious... No!

Then what to do?

Well, for starters, stop stretching them.

Then, simply reverse your pattern of "arms down" to the pattern of "arms up" as often as 3–4 times daily. This will give these muscles a needed break, and hopefully relieve some tension buildup.

What is the "arms up" pattern?

Any position where your arms are raised up alongside your ears:

- Lie down on your back and rest (knees bent or straight) with arms up.

- Hang on a horizontal bar, or hook your fingers on a door frame for a few breaths.

- Bend forward and let the arms hang loose for a minute.

- Take the Child's Pose (in yoga) and rest for a minute.

Some or all of these poses should be practiced if you experience the crunchy spots, achy-ness, regular tension, and sharp and shooting nerve sensations in your shoulders and neck.

Why do these positions work?

Because they slack those over-stretched muscles. They give them a break.

What else can we do instead of stretching?

The best thing to do for any muscle is to keep it strong. Strength is the long-term solution. Strong muscles do not tire easily and are able to sustain longer loading.

Second best, or perhaps as important as strength, is to get a massage, or find a way to apply pressure to relieve tension. Pressure should be applied on a regular basis to all the problematic areas with the intention of soothing and *smoothing out* the stringy, knotty, crunchy spots so they do not have a chance to become chronic.

Article 5: Treating pain and tension in the mid-back

Pain and tightness in the mid-back and between the scapulae (shoulder blades) is a common condition that massage therapists see on a daily basis.

It seems that almost everyone is feeling a degree of strain in that area. Let's take a look at what's happening and how we can help release it on our own, and with massage.

First of all, this area is one busy intersection of muscles and other tissues (**Diagram 58**).

Many layers of muscle tissue

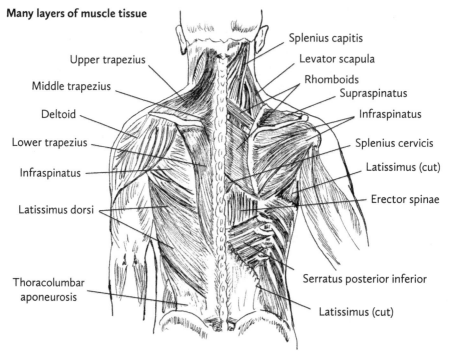

Diagram 58. Major back muscles

Busy intersection means many layers—muscles over muscles at different angles. For example, rhomboids and the lower trapezius crisscross each other at an almost exact right angle, and both attach at the medial border of the scapula (**Diagram 58**).

These crisscross spots are the typical points of pain. Often, such muscle layers get "glued" to each other in these spots, limiting movement and restricting blood flow.

In addition, the middle of our back is the least mobile area thanks to the ribcage. The ribcage protects internal organs and restricts mobility of the mid-back compared to the neck and the lower back. This lack of mobility further limits the blood flow to all of these muscle layers.

However, to make matters worse, the biggest contributors to pain and tension in the mid-back and between the scapulae are postural and habitual patterns:

- Poor posture due to general weakness of the muscles of the mid-back (rhomboids, trapezius, infraspinatus).

- Sitting too much with the back rounded (in a "C-curve").

- Sleeping in the side position makes these muscles over-stretched and often "torn off" the medial border of the scapula.

Diagram 59 shows the infamous Upper Cross syndrome. Notice the weak muscles of the mid-back: the lower trapezius and serratus anterior. We can add to this list rhomboids, the erector spinae, and infraspinatus.

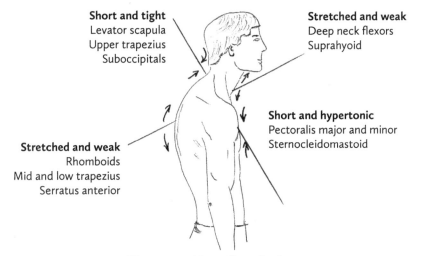

Short and tight
Levator scapula
Upper trapezius
Suboccipitals

Stretched and weak
Deep neck flexors
Suprahyoid

Short and hypertonic
Pectoralis major and minor
Sternocleidomastoid

Stretched and weak
Rhomboids
Mid and low trapezius
Serratus anterior

Diagram 59. Upper Cross Syndrome

What to do

1. Do not stretch your mid-back. It's already overstretched!

2. Instead, strengthen it with Cobra Pose, and Superman/Woman Pose.

3. Prop your arm on a side pillow if you sleep on your side. Change your sleeping position to supine, or half-side-half-supine, so that the back is not rounded while sleeping, and the area between the shoulder blades is not stretched but slacked.

4. Put some pressure on it! Use a golf ball, a massage tool, or even the corner of a doorframe. Pressure relieves tension—that is what massage is for!

5. Roll up a blanket and lie down over it. Place it across and under your shoulder blades. Rest there for about a minute. In this position, the muscles are slacked (the opposite of stretched). This is positional release, which is the reverse of the rounded "C-curve" position we often get from sitting too long. Our brain must receive the "slacked muscle" messages.

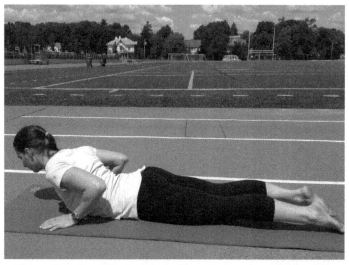

Ginger Howell, professional triathlete, demonstrates Cobra Pose

6. Last, but not least, get a massage if you experience this kind of pain and discomfort. Deep bodywork will break up the "glued-up" spots, flush them out with blood supply, and jumpstart the return of the healthy-feeling muscles.

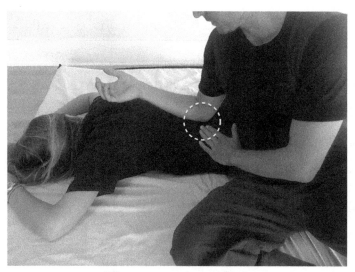

Elbow compressions on back

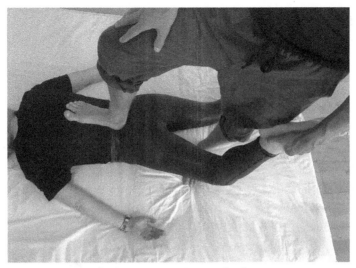

Foot compressions on back
Sometimes, the elbow is not enough

About the Author

Slava Kolpakov, originally from Krasnoyarsk, a city in Siberia, Russia, is a neuromuscular therapist, Thai Massage instructor, yoga philosophy teacher, and author. Slava grew up in the Soviet Union with yoga-practicing parents and has been teaching yoga, breathwork, and meditation since 2002.

Slava has studied and practiced Thai Massage in the United States and Thailand since 2006. He received his Massage Therapy training in 2005 in San Diego at the International Professional School of Bodywork.

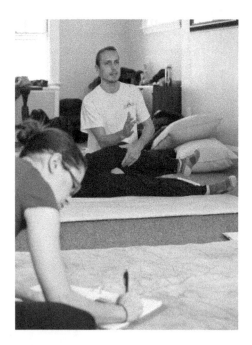

From 2007 to 2018, Slava owned and operated the East West Massage Center in Boston, MA, a massage clinic with 20 massage therapists and two locations. He and his massage teams have worked with elite and Olympic athletes around New England, with Harvard, Yale, and Columbia Universities' sports teams.

Slava's experience is in combining clinical work such as Neuromuscular Therapy (NMT) with traditional Thai Massage, and in helping people prevent and treat injuries. He resides in San Diego, CA, with his wife and son, and teaches Thai Neuromuscular Massage at the International College of Holistic Studies and internationally.

Bibliography

Baker, J. (2003) *Intro to NMT* [self-published].

Baker, J. (2012) *Musculoskeletal Anatomy Layer by Layer*. Apple Books. Available at: https://books.apple.com/us/book/musculoskeletal-anatomy/id539817408

Biel, A. (2001) *Trail Guide to the Body* (2nd Edition). Books of Discovery.

Cyriax, J.H. (1982) *Textbook of Orthopaedic Medicine, Volume One: Diagnosis of Soft Tissue Lesions*. Baillière Tindall.

Cyriax, J.H. (1984) *Textbook of Orthopaedic Medicine, Volume Two: Treatment by Manipulation, Massage and Injection*. Baillière Tindall.

Ellis, A., Wiseman, N., and Boss, K. (1991) *Fundamentals of Chinese Acupuncture*. Paradigm Publications.

Gold, R. (2006) *Thai Massage: A Traditional Medical Technique* (2nd Edition). Mosby.

Simons, D.G. Travell, J.G., and Simons, L.S. (1998) *Travell & Simons' Myofascial Pain and Dysfunction: The Trigger Point Manual*, (2nd Edition). Baltimore, MD: Lippincott Williams & Wilkins.

Index